New Jersey EMS FIELD GUIDE

NEW JERSEY DEPARTMENT of HEALTH and SENIOR SERVICES

World Headquarters

Jones & Bartlett Learning	Jones & Bartlett Learning Canada	Jones & Bartlett Learning International
5 Wall Street	6339 Ormindale Way	The Exchange
Burlington, MA 01803	Mississauga, Ontario L5V 1J2	Express Park
978-443-5000	Canada	Bristol Road
info@jblearning.com		Bridgewater TA6 4RR
www.jblearning.com		United Kingdom

Jones & Bartlett Learning books and products are available through most bookstores and online booksellers. To contact Jones & Bartlett Learning directly, call 800-832-0034, fax 978-443-8000, or visit our website, www.jblearning.com.

Substantial discounts on bulk quantities of Jones & Bartlett Learning publications are available to corporations, professional associations, and other qualified organizations. For details and specific discount information, contact the special sales department at Jones & Bartlett Learning via the above contact information or send an email to specialsales@jblearning.com.

particular situation, because circumstances and the patient's physical condition can vary widely from one emergency to another. Nor is it intended that this field guide shall in any way advise emergency personnel concerning legal authority to perform the activities or procedures discussed. Such determinations should be made only with the aid of legal counsel.

Production Credits

Publisher: Kimberly Brophy
Director, Public Safety Group—Matthew Maniscalco
Acquisitions Editor—EMS: Christine Emerton
Associate Managing Editor: Amanda J. Green
Senior Production Editor: Susan Schultz
Director of Marketing: Alisha Weisman
VP, Manufacturing and Inventory Control: Therese Connell
Text Design: Anne Spencer
Cover Design: Scott Moden
Photo Research Coordinator: Jessica Elias
Composition: Shepherd, Inc.
Algorithm Development: Bill Porter
Algorithm Illustration: DiacriTech
Illustration: PD&PS, Inc.
Printing and Binding: Transcontinental
Cover Printing: Transcontinental
Photo Credits: EMSC Bear: Courtesy of the Emergency Medical Services for Children National Resource Center; Chapter 5, page 218 (top) © Dr. P. Marazzi/Photo Researchers, Inc.; page 221 (bottom) © Sebarnes/Dreamstime.com; Chapter 6, page 288 (top) © Jaimie Duplass/ShutterStock, Inc.; page 289 (top) © Cate Frost/ShutterStock, Inc.; Unless otherwise indicated, all photographs and illustrations are under copyright of Jones & Bartlett Learning or have been provided by the authors.

ISBN: 978-0-7637-9864-2

6048
Printed in Canada
15 14 13 12 11 10 9 8 7 6 5 4 3 2 1

How to Use the Field Guide

The algorithms contained in the field guide are color-coded according to the level of provider that should perform the task. White boxes within algorithms apply to BLS providers and red boxes apply to ALS providers.

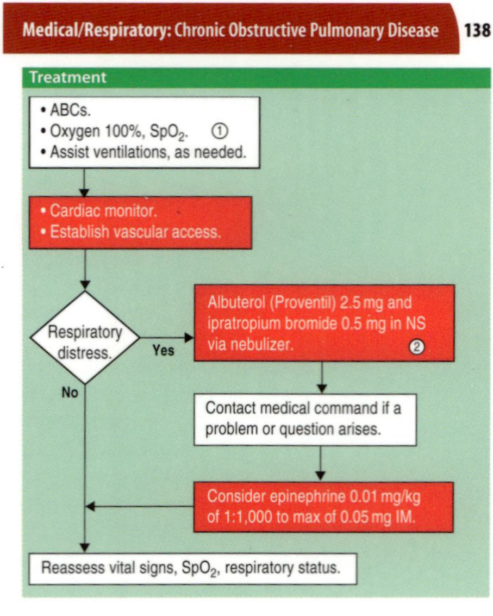

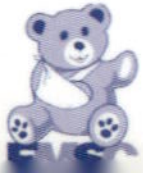

Special considerations for the pediatric population are included as necessary and are identifiable by the Emergency Medical Services for Children (EMSC) bear.

Acknowledgements

The New Jersey Department of Health and Senior Services (NJDHSS) Office of Emergency Medical Services (OEMS) acknowledges the following individuals and organizations for their assistance in developing this BLS/ALS Field Guide:

Mary E. O'Dowd, MPH, Commissioner, NJ Dept. of Health & Senior Services

Christina Tan, MD, MPH, Deputy Commissioner, NJ Dept. of Health & Senior Services

Christopher R. Rinn, Assistant Commissioner, NJ Dept. of Health & Senior Services

Members of the NJ EMS Advisory Council

Jennifer Waxler, DO, Chairperson

Members of the NJ EMSC Advisory Council

Alfred Sacchetti, Jr., MD, Chairperson

Members of the NJ MICU Advisory Council

Mark Merlin, DO, Chairperson

NJ Office of Emergency Medical Services Staff

Karen Halupke, Director

Steven Cohen, NREMT-P, Jersey City Medical Center

Howard Felderman, MD, Chilton Hospital

Bryan Fischberg, NREMT-P, RWJ-University Hospital

Nancy Kelly-Goodstein, NJ MICP, NJ Office of Emergency Medical Services

Andy Lovell, NREMT-P, Gloucester County Emergency Medical Service

Kathleen Lutz, CPNP, NJ Office of Emergency Medical Services

Steven M. Marcus, MD, NJ Poison Information & Education System

Gerard McEntee, NJ MICP, NJ State First Aid Council

Christopher Ryan, NREMT-P, NJ Office of Emergency Medical Services

Stephen Vetrano, DO, Chair NJ BLS Subcommittee & NJ EMT Training Fund Council

Section 1 General Information 2

Assessment Tools 2
Communication 21
Documentation 24
Infection Control and Standard Precautions 26
Patient Confidentiality and HIPAA 28
Social Media Tips 29
Patient Refusal 30
Requesting an Air Medical Unit 32
Requesting BLS/ALS 34

Section 2 Medical Treatment 35

Medical 35

Abdominal Pain, Nausea, and/or Vomiting 35
Abuse and Neglect 38
Allergic Reactions and Anaphylaxis 44
Altered Mental Status 48
Behavioral Emergencies and Psychiatric Disorders 51
Diabetic Emergencies 55
Frostbite 58
Hypoperfusion: Nontraumatic Shock 60
Hyperthermia 63
Hypothermia 66
Near Drowning 70
Pain Management 73
Seizures 76
Stroke and Cerebrovascular Accidents 79

Cardiac Emergencies 82
Chest Pain and Acute Myocardial Infarction 82
CPR Guidelines 87
Pediatric Cardiac Arrest 90
Pediatric Bradycardia 92
Pediatric Tachycardia 93

Advanced Cardiac Life Support 95
Asystole and Pulseless Electrical Activity 95
Bradycardia 97
Ventricular Fibrillation and Pulseless Ventricular Tachycardia 99
Narrow Complex Tachycardia—Stable 102
Narrow Complex Tachycardia—Unstable 104
Ventricular Tachycardia with Pulses—Stable 107
Ventricular Tachycardia with Pulses—Unstable 108

Obstetrical Emergencies 110
Normal Delivery Childbirth 110
Abnormal Delivery Childbirth 114
Pregnancy Bleeding 119
Neonatal Resuscitation 122

Overdose/Poisoning 126
CNS Depressant 126
Tricyclic Antidepressant 129

Respiratory Distress 132
Asthma 132
Chronic Obstructive Pulmonary Disease 135
Congestive Heart Failure 138
Croup and Epiglottitis 141
Obstructed Airway 144

Section 3 Trauma Treatment 149

Amputation 149
Burns 152
Eye Injuries 157
General Management of Trauma 160
Head and Spine Injuries 163
Orthopedic Injuries 166
Soft Tissue Injuries 170
Transport Guidelines 174

Section 4 Procedures 178

Cricothyrotomy 178
Epinephrine Auto-Injector 182
Intraosseous Infusion 184
Intubation Checklist 187
Oxygen Administration 191
ST-Segment Elevation Myocardial Infarction (STEMI) 192
Stroke Assessment 195
Tension Pneumothorax Decompression 197
Ventricular Assist Devices 200

Section 5 Emergency Preparedness 202

Emergency Preparedness Definitions 202
EMS Task Force 203
Hazardous Materials 207
Mass Casualty Incident 213
NJ Burn Matrix for Mass Casualties 222
Personal Protective Equipment 224
Terrorism and Weapons of Mass Destruction 233
Cyanide Exposure and Treatment 241
Organophosphate Exposure 245

Section 6 Miscellaneous 249

Anatomy References 249
Dermatome Chart 253
Common Medical Abbreviations 254
Communication Flipchart 259
Developmental Disabilities 271
Death of a Patient 275
Do Not Resuscitate Orders 277
Heat Index/Wind Chill Charts 280
Measurement Conversions 282
Medical Spanish 286
Medications 290
New Jersey Poison Information and Education System 309
Phone Numbers and Radio Frequencies 312
Stress Management 322
Vehicle Safety Reminders 325

Assessment Tools

Patient Assessment

The assessment process is divided into five main parts:

1. Scene size-up
2. Primary assessment
3. History taking
4. Secondary assessment
5. Reassessment

Patient assessment is divided into components to encourage an organized approach, but it needs to be flexible to the patient and to the situation.

Scene Size-up
- Ensure scene safety
- Determine mechanism of injury/nature of illness
- Take standard precautions
- Determine number of patients
- Consider additional/specialized resources

↓

Primary Assessment
- Form a general impression
- Assess level of consciousness
- Assess the airway: identify and treat life threats
- Assess breathing: identify and treat life threats
- Assess circulation: identify and treat life threats
- Perform rapid scan
- Determine priority of patient care and transport

↓

History Taking:
- Investigate the chief complaint (history of present illness)
- Obtain SAMPLE history

Secondary Assessment: Medical
- Assess vital signs using the appropriate monitoring device
- Systematically assess the patient
  - Full-body scan and/or focused assessment

Secondary Assessment: Trauma
- Assess vital signs using the appropriate monitoring device
- Systematically assess the patient
  - Full-body scan and/or focused assessment

Reassessment
- Repeat the primary assessment
- Reassess vital signs
- Reassess the chief complaint
- Recheck interventions
- Identify and treat changes in the patient's condition
- Reassess patient
  - Unstable patients: every 5 minutes
  - Stable patients: every 15 minutes

A variety of helpful assessment tools may be used throughout the patient assessment process. Some of the more common assessment tools are discussed in this section.

Glasgow Coma Scale

The Glasgow Coma Scale (GCS) score can be helpful in providing information on patients with changes in mental status. When you are reporting the GCS score, you should document or report each section (i.e., Eye opening: 3, Verbal response: 4, Motor response: 5 = GCS score of 12) to document baseline function in each area. **Table 1** shows guidelines for determining the GCS.

TABLE 1 Glasgow Coma Scale

Activity	Score	Adult
Eye opening	4	Spontaneously
	3	To command
	2	To pain
	1	No response
Best verbal response	5	Oriented
	4	Confused
	3	Inappropriate words
	2	Incomprehensible
	1	No response
Best motor response	6	Obeys command
	5	Localizes pain
	4	Withdraws from pain
	3	Flexion (decorticate)
	2	Extension (decerebrate)
	1	No response

Score 13–15: May indicate mild dysfunction, although a person with no neurologic disabilities would receive a GCS of 15.
Score 9–12: May indicate moderate dysfunction.
Score 3–8: Is indicative of severe dysfunction.

Vital Signs

Table 2 shows guidelines for adult vital signs.

TABLE 2 Vital Signs

	Heart Rate (beats/min)	Respirations (breaths/min)	Blood Pressure (systolic mm Hg)
Adult	60–100	12–20	90–140

OPQRST

The mnemonic OPQRST (see **Table 3**) can be very helpful in the assessment of pain.

TABLE 3 OPQRST

Onset	When did the problem begin and what caused it?
Provocation or **P**alliation	Does anything make it feel better or worse? How are you most comfortable?
Quality	What is the pain like? Is it sharp, dull, crushing, or tearing? Ask the patient to describe the pain.
Region/Radiation	Where does it hurt? Does the pain move anywhere?
Severity	On a scale of 1 to 10, how would you rate your pain?
Timing	Has the pain been constant, or does it come and go? How long have you had the pain (often answered under "O," onset)? When did the pain start?

SAMPLE History

SAMPLE history, a mnemonic used to gather a general past medical or trauma history, assists you in gathering important information from the patient. Use the mnemonic SAMPLE to obtain the following information:

- S **Signs and symptoms:** What signs and symptoms occurred at the onset of the incident? Does the patient report pain?
- A **Allergies:** Is the patient allergic to any medication, food, or other substance? What reactions did the patient have to any of them? If the patient has no known allergies, you should note this on the patient care report as "no known allergies" or "NKA."
- M **Medications:** What medication is the patient prescribed? What dosage is prescribed? How often does the patient take the medication? What prescriptions, over-the-counter medications, or herbal medications has the patient taken in the last 12 hours? This includes medications taken for birth control or erectile dysfunction. How much was taken and when? Does the patient take recreational drugs or drink alcohol?
- P **Pertinent past medical history:** Does the patient have any history of medical, surgical, or trauma occurrences? Has the patient had a recent illness or injury, fall, or blow to the head? Is there important family history that should be known?
- L **Last oral intake:** When did the patient last eat or drink? What did the patient eat or drink, and how much was consumed? Did the patient take any drugs or drink alcohol? Has there been any other oral intake in the last 4 hours?
- E **Events leading up to the injury or illness:** What are the key events that led up to this incident? What occurred between the onset of the incident and your arrival? What was the patient doing when this illness started? What was the patient doing when this injury happened?

DCAP-BTLS

The mnemonic DCAP-BTLS will help remind you what to look for when inspecting and palpating various body regions. Each area of the body is evaluated for the following:

D Deformities

C Contusions

A Abrasions

P Punctures/Penetrations

B Burns

T Tenderness

L Lacerations

S Swelling

The Wong-Baker FACES Scale

Pain scales using pictures of facial expressions, such as the Wong-Baker FACES Scale, may be helpful in assessing the patient's level of pain.

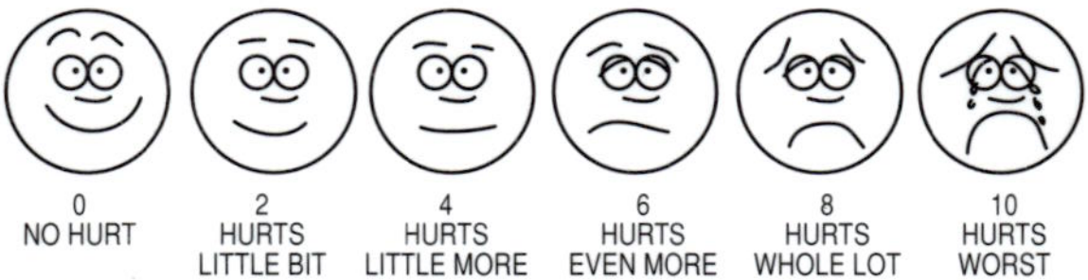

From Hockenberry MJ, Wilson D, Wikelstein ML. *Wong's Essentials of Pediatric Nursing,* ed. 7, St. Louis, 2005, p. 1259. Used with permission. Copyright, Mosby.

PEARRL

The letters PEARRL serve as a useful guide in assessing the pupils. They stand for the following:

P Pupils

E Equal

A And

R Round

R Regular in size

L react to Light

Revised Trauma Score

Several different trauma scoring systems are available. The one that is the most commonly used for patients with head trauma is the Revised Trauma Score (RTS), because it is heavily weighted to compensate for major head injury without multisystem injury or major physiologic changes.

The RTS is a physiologic scoring system that is also used to assess the severity of a trauma patient's injuries. Objective data used to calculate the RTS includes the Glasgow Coma Scale (GCS) score, systolic blood pressure (SBP), and respiratory rate (RR). In addition to assessing injury severity, the RTS has also demonstrated reliability in predicting survival in patients with severe injuries. The highest RTS a patient can receive is 12; the lowest is 0. The RTS is calculated as shown in **Table 4**.

TABLE 4 Revised Trauma Score

GCS	SBP	RR	Value
13–15	> 89 mm Hg	10–29 breaths/min	4
9–12	76–89 mm Hg	> 29 breaths/min	3
6–8	50–75 mm Hg	6–9 breaths/min	2
4–5	1–49 mm Hg	1–5 breaths/min	1
3	0	0	0

Burns: Palmar Method

The Palmar Method is a means of assessing the total body surface area (TBSA) burned. This assessment uses the size of the patient's hand (including the fingers) to represent about 1% of the patient's body surface area.

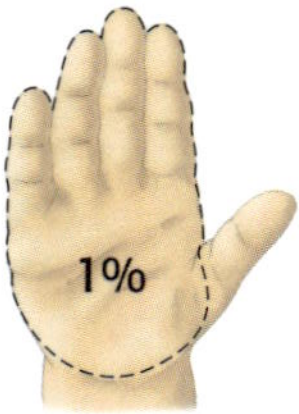

Burns: The Rule of 9's

The Rule of 9's is another quick way to estimate the amount of body surface area that has been burned on a patient. The Rule of 9's divides the body into sections, each of which is approximately 9% of the total body surface area.

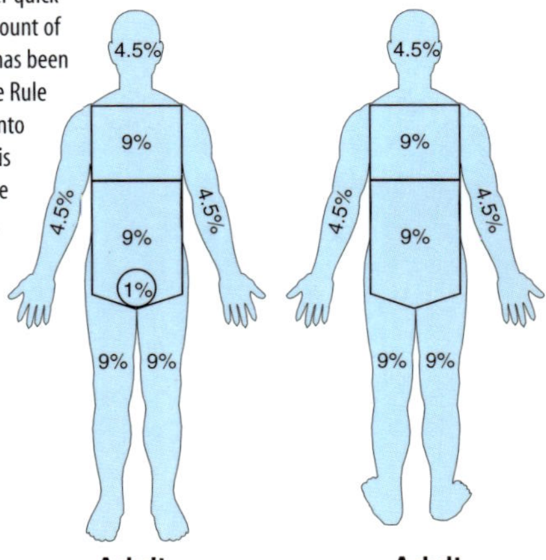

Adult (front)

Adult (back)

Stroke Assessment

Many EMS services use the Cincinnati Prehospital Stroke Scale (**Table 5**) or the Los Angeles Prehospital Stroke Screen (**Table 6**) to rapidly identify the stroke patient in the field.

TABLE 5 Cincinnati Prehospital Stroke Scale

Test	Normal	Abnormal
Facial droop: Ask patient to show teeth or smile.	Both sides of face move equally well.	One side of face does not move as well as other.
Arm drift: Ask patient to close eyes and hold both arms out with palms up.	Both arms move the same, or both arms do not move.	One arm does not move, or one arm drifts down compared with the other side.
Speech: Ask patient to say, "The sky is blue in Cincinnati."	Patient uses correct words with no slurring.	Patient slurs words, uses inappropriate words, or is unable to speak.

TABLE 6 Los Angeles Prehospital Stroke Screen

Criteria	Yes	Unknown	No
1. Age > 45 years.	☐	☐	☐
2. History of seizures or epilepsy absent.	☐	☐	☐
3. Symptoms < 24 hours.	☐	☐	☐
4. At baseline, patient is not wheelchair-bound or bedridden.	☐	☐	☐
5. Blood glucose is between 60–400 mg/dL.	☐	☐	☐
6. Obvious asymmetry (right versus left) in any of the following three exam categories (must be unilateral).	☐	☐	☐

	Equal	Right Weak	Left Weak
Facial smile/grimace	☐	☐ Droop	☐ Droop
Grip	☐	☐ Weak grip ☐ No grip	☐ Weak grip ☐ No grip
Arm strength	☐	☐ Drifts down ☐ Falls rapidly	☐ Drifts down ☐ Falls rapidly

Note: If criteria 1–6 are marked yes, the probability of a stroke is 97%.

Pediatric Assessment

Pediatric Vital Signs

	Heart Rate (beats/min)	Respirations (breaths/min)	Blood Pressure (systolic mm Hg)
Adolescent (13+ yrs)	60–100	12–16	> 90
School age (6–12 years)	70–120	18–30	> 80
Preschool age (3–5 years)	80–140	22–34	> 75
Toddler (1–3 years)	90–150	24–40	> 70*
Infants (1 month to 1 year)	100–160	30–60	> 60*
Newborn/neonate (0–1 month)	100–160	30–60	> 60*

* Infants and children 3 years or younger: evaluate the central pulses instead of measuring blood pressure.

The Wong-Baker FACES Scale

In older children, pain scales using pictures of facial expressions, such as the Wong-Baker FACES Scale, may be helpful in assessing the pediatric patient's level of pain.

From Hockenberry MJ, Wilson D, Wikelstein ML. *Wong's Essentials of Pediatric Nursing*, ed. 7, St. Louis,

Pediatric Assessment Triangle

The pediatric assessment triangle (PAT) is a structured assessment tool that allows you to rapidly form a general impression of the pediatric patient's condition without touching him or her. It provides a "first glance" assessment to identify the general category of the pediatric patient's physiologic problem and to establish urgency for treatment and/or transport. The PAT is a 15- to 30-second visual assessment of the pediatric patient.

The PAT consists of three elements: appearance (muscle tone and mental status), work of breathing, and circulation to the skin. The only equipment required for the PAT is your own eyes and ears; no stethoscope, blood pressure cuff, cardiac monitor, or pulse oximeter is required.

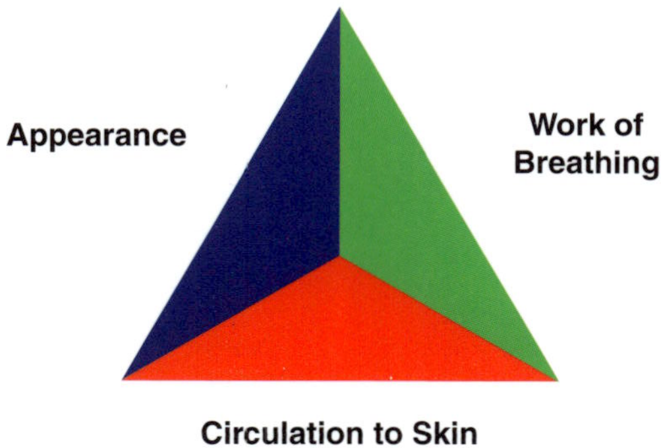

Pediatric Glasgow Coma Scale (GCS)

The Pediatric Glasgow Coma Scale (**Table 7**) can be used to assess the pediatric patient's level of consciousness.

TABLE 7 Pediatric Glasgow Coma Scale

Activity	Score	Infant (0–12 mo)	Score	Child (1+ yr)
Eye opening	4	Spontaneously	4	Spontaneously
	3	To speech	3	To command
	2	To pain	2	To pain
	1	No response	1	No response
Best verbal response	5	Coos, babbles	5	Oriented
	4	Irritable, cries	4	Confused
	3	Cries to pain	3	Inappropriate words
	2	Moans, grunts	2	Incomprehensible
	1	No response	1	No response
Best motor response	6	Spontaneous	6	Obeys command
	5	Localizes pain	5	Localizes pain
	4	Withdraws from pain	4	Withdraws from pain
	3	Flexion (decorticate)	3	Flexion (decorticate)
	2	Extension (decerebrate)	2	Extension (decerebrate)
	1	No response	1	No response

Score 13–15: May indicate mild dysfunction, although a person with no neurologic disabilities would receive a GCS of 15.

Score 9–12: May indicate moderate dysfunction.

Score 3–8: Is indicative of severe dysfunction.

APGAR Scoring System

The APGAR score is the standard scoring system used to assess the activity status of a newborn at 1-, 5-, and 10-minute intervals after birth. This system assigns a number value (0, 1, or 2) to five areas of activity (**Table 8**).

TABLE 8 APGAR Score

	Score		
Area of Activity	**2**	**1**	**0**
Appearance	Entire infant is pink.	Body is pink, but hands and feet remain blue.	Entire infant is blue or pale.
Pulse	> 100 beats/min.	< 100 beats/min.	Absent pulse.
Grimace or irritability	Infant cries and tries to move foot away from finger snapped against sole of foot.	Infant gives a weak cry in response to stimulus.	Infant does not cry or react to stimulus.
Activity or muscle tone	Infant resists attempts to straighten hips and knees.	Infant makes weak attempts to resist straightening.	Infant is completely limp, with no muscle tone.
Respiration	Rapid respirations.	Slow respirations.	Absent respirations.

Pediatric Burns: The Palmar Method

The Palmar Method uses the size of the patient's hand (including the fingers) to represent about 1% of the patient's body surface area.

Pediatric Burns: The Rule of 9's

The Rule of 9's can also be used during a pediatric assessment to estimate the amount of surface area that has been burned. Burns to children are generally considered more serious than burns to adults. Infants and children have more surface area relative to their total body mass, which means greater fluid and heat loss. Children also do not tolerate burns as well as adults do. Children are more likely to go into shock, develop hypothermia, and experience airway problems. An infant's or child's hand is approximately 1% of its total body area. The adolescent burn chart is the same as the adult burn chart. Refer back to the adult section for those numbers.

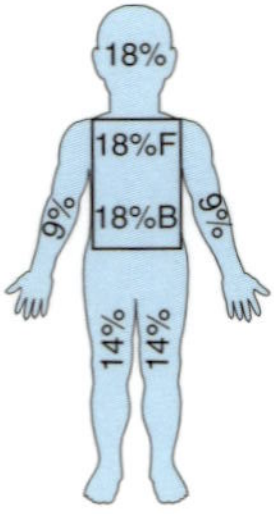

Infant

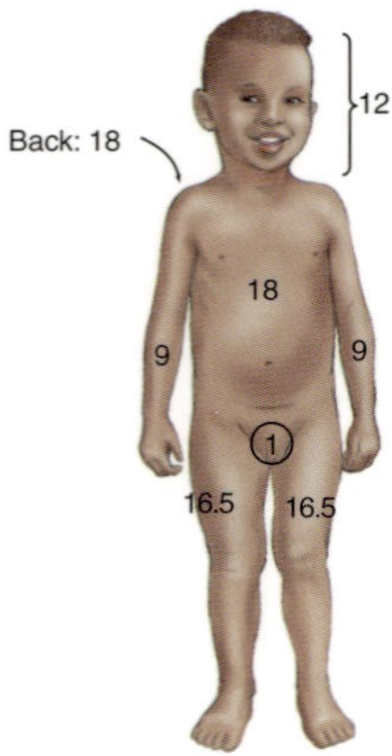

Child

Equipment Size

The best way to identify the appropriately sized equipment for a pediatric patient is to use the pediatric resuscitation tape measure (e.g., Broselow Tape®), which can determine weight as well as height in pediatric patients weighing up to 75 lbs (34 kg).

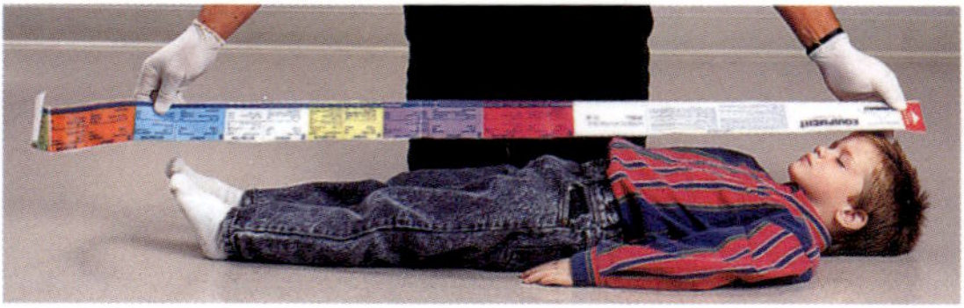

TABLE 9 Airway, Breathing, Circulation Equipment Sizes

Age and Weight (kg)	Airway and Breathing			Circulation	
	O_2 Mask	Oral Airways	Bag-Valve Mask	Suction	BP Cuff
Premie 1–1.5 kg	Premie Newborn	Infant	Infant	6–8F	Premie Newborn
Newborn 0–6 mos 3.5–7.5 kg	Newborn	Infant Small	Infant	8F	Newborn Infant
6–12 mos 7.5 – 10 kg	Pediatric	Small	Pediatric	8-10F	Infant Child
1–3 yrs 10–15 kg	Pediatric	Small	Pediatric	10F	Child
4–7 yrs 17.5–23 kg	Pediatric	Medium	Pediatric	14F	Child
$\geq$ 8 yrs $\geq$ 25 kg	Adult	Medium Large	Pediatric Adult	14F	Child Adult

Newborn Resuscitation

Dry, Warm, Position, Suction, Tactile stimulation.

If respirations < 40 or heart rate < 80 or central cyanosis:
Administer blow-by O_2.

If no change and airway is clear:
Administer 100% O_2 via BVM at
40–60 breaths/min.
Request ALS.

If no increase in heart rate
after 15–30 sec of BVM
resuscitation:
Chest compressions
at 120/min.
Continue
ventilations.

Geriatric Assessment

The GEMS Diamond

The GEMS diamond was created to help you remember what is different about the older patient. The GEMS diamond is not intended to be a format for the approach to geriatric patients, nor is it intended to replace the ABCs of care. Instead, it serves as an acronym for the issues to be considered when assessing every older patient.

G Geriatric Patients

- Present atypically
- Deserve respect
- Experience normal changes with age

E Environmental Assessment

- Check for hazardous conditions that may be present (eg, poor wiring, rotted floors, unventilated gas heaters, broken window glass, clutter that prevents adequate egress).
- Are smoke detectors present and working? Is carbon monoxide present?
- Is the home too hot or too cold?
- Is there an odor of feces or urine in the home? Is bedding soiled?
- Is food present in the home? Is it adequate and unspoiled?
- Are liquor bottles present? If so, are they lying empty?
- If the patient has a disability, are appropriate assistive devices (eg, ramps, rails, wheelchairs, or walkers) present?
- Does the patient have access to a telephone?
- Are medications out of date or unmarked, or are prescriptions for the same or similar medications from many physicians? Are any of the medications prescribed to other people?
- If living with others, is the patient confined to one part of the home?
- If the patient is residing in a nursing facility, does the care appear to be adequate to meet the patient's needs?

continues

The GEMS Diamond, continued

M Medical Assessment

- Older patients tend to have a variety of medical problems, making assessment more complex. Keep this in mind in all cases—both trauma and medical. A trauma patient may have an underlying medical condition that could have caused or may be exacerbated by the injury.
- Obtaining a medical history is important in older patients, regardless of the chief complaint.
- Primary assessment
- Reassessment

S Social Assessment

- Assess activities of daily living (eating, dressing, bathing, toileting).
- Are these activities being provided for the patient? If so, by whom?
- Are there delays in obtaining food, medication, or other necessary items? The patient may complain of this, or the environment may suggest this.
- If in an institutional setting, is the patient able to feed himself or herself? If not, is food still sitting on the food tray? Has the patient been lying in his or her own urine or feces for prolonged periods?
- Does the patient have a social network? Does the patient have a mechanism to interact socially with others on a daily basis?

Communication

Therapeutic Communication

Therapeutic communication uses various communication techniques and strategies to encourage patients to express how they are feeling and to allow the responder to achieve a positive relationship with the patient.

TABLE 1 Factors and Strategies to Consider During Communication

- Age
- Body language
- Clothing
- Culture
- Educational background
- Environment
- Eye contact
- Facial expression
- Gender
- Posture
- Voice tempo
- Volume

Verbal Communication

TABLE 2 Guidelines for Verbal Communication

- Introduce yourself.
- Ask the patient's name and use it.
- Make and keep eye contact.
- Use language the patient understands.
- Speak slowly, clearly, and distinctly.
- Tell the truth.
- Allow time for the patient to respond.
- Limit the number of people talking with the patient.
- Be aware of body language.
- Act and speak in a calm, confident manner.
- Respect cultural norms.
- Use open- and close-ended questions appropriately.
- Treat all patients as if they were a member of your family.

Radio Communications

The principal reason for radio communication is to facilitate communication between you, dispatch, medical command, and/or other responders.

TABLE 3 Tips for Radio Communication

- Ensure a clear frequency before speaking.
- To speak, use the "press to talk" button and wait 1 second before speaking.
- Hold the microphone 2 to 3 inches from your mouth.
- Address the unit you are calling and provide the name of your unit.
- The unit you call will signal that you can begin your transmission.
- Use a clear, calm, and steady voice and speak at a reasonable pace.
- Keep the transmission brief.
- Use clear text.
- Avoid the use of codes or agency-specific terms.
- Do not use useless or meaningless phrases, such as "Be advised."
- Limit saying "please," "thank you," and "you're welcome."
- When transmitting numbers, such as an address, provide both the number and the individual digits, for example, "Respond to 381, 3-8-1, South Main Street."
- Remember that the airwaves are public and the use of scanners is popular.
- Remain objective and impartial in describing patients.
- Never use profanity.
- Use the words "affirmative" and "negative" instead of "yes" or "no."
- Use the standard format for transmission of information.
- When you are finished transmitting, indicate this by saying "over."
- Use EMS frequencies only for EMS communication.
- Monitor background noise.
- Do not use names; protect the privacy of patients.

Communicating with Other Health Care Professionals

The easiest way to verbally report your findings is to use the same systematic approach you follow during the patient assessment process. You may have to transfer care of a patient to another professional face to face or you may have to provide an oral report over the radio. The following list contains the essential elements that need to be communicated:

1. Provide unit identity and level of care.
2. Provide the age and gender of the patient.
3. Describe the history of the incident.
4. Describe the patient's chief complaint.
5. Describe the patient's level of responsiveness.
6. Describe how you found the patient.
7. Report the status of the patient's vital signs, airway, breathing, and circulation (including severe bleeding).
8. Describe the results of the physical examination.
9. Report any pertinent medical conditions using the SAMPLE (Signs and symptoms, Allergies, Medications, Pertinent past history, Last oral intake, and Events leading to injury or illness) format.
10. Report the interventions provided and how the patient responded to them.

Documentation

Patient Care Report

The patient care report (PCR), also known as a prehospital care report, is the legal document used to record all aspects of the care your patient received, from initial dispatch to arrival at the hospital. You will most likely use one of two types of forms:

- Traditional written form
- Computerized version of form (ePCR)*

*The ePCR system is available through the NJ Department of Health and Senior Services. For more information visit www.state.nj.us/health/ems.

TABLE 1 Sample Components of a Patient Care Report

• Patient's name, gender, date of birth, and address	• Time of the call
• Dispatched as (when the ambulance was called and the nature of the call as reported by the dispatcher)	• Location of the call
• Chief complaint	• Time of dispatch
• Location of the patient when first seen (including specific details, especially if the incident is a motor vehicle crash or when criminal activity is suspected)	• Time of arrival at the scene
• Rescue and treatment given before your arrival	• Time of leaving the scene
• Signs and symptoms found during your patient assessment	• Time of arrival at the hospital

• Care and treatment given by you at the site and during transport	• Patient's insurance information
• Vital signs	• Names and/or certification numbers of the EMTs who responded to the call
• SAMPLE history	• Name of the base hospital involved in the call
• Changes in vital signs and condition	
• Date of the call	• Type of call to the scene: emergency or routine

TABLE 2 Guidelines for Proper Documentation

• Fill in all boxes completely.	• If you accidently leave out information, create an addendum to the report.
• Ensure accuracy of information.	• Document refusal of care and have the patient sign the form.
• Avoid drawing conclusions.	• Document medical advice given to the patient.
• Present facts based on findings.	• Document the care you wish to provide.
• Use standard abbreviations only.	• Draw a single line through an error, initial it, and write the correct information next to the error.
• Spell words correctly.	
• Record the time for all findings.	

Infection Control and Standard Precautions

Standard precautions are intended to reduce the risk of transmission of bloodborne and other pathogens from both recognized and unrecognized sources. They are the basic level of infection-control precautions. Standard precautions must be used in the care of all patients.

Hand hygiene: Wash hands for 20 seconds with soap and water, especially if visibly soiled. Clean hands with alcohol-based hand rub if not visibly soiled. Wash hands before and after any direct patient contact; between patients; immediately after gloves are removed; before handling an invasive device; after touching blood, body fluids, secretions, excretions, non-intact skin, and contaminated items; during patient care; and when moving from a contaminated to a clean body site on the patient.

Gloves: Wear when touching blood, body fluids, secretions, excretions, mucous membranes, and non-intact skin. Change between tasks and procedures on the same patient after contact with potentially infectious material. Remove after use, before touching noncontaminated items or surfaces, and before going to another patient. Perform hand hygiene immediately after removal of gloves.

Gown: Wear during procedures when the caregiver's clothing/exposed skin may be exposed to blood, body fluids, secretions, excretions, or contaminated items.

Mask, eye protection: Wear during procedures likely to generate splashes or sprays of blood, body fluids, secretions, or excretions.

Needles and other sharp objects: Do not recap, bend, break, or hand manipulate used needles. Use needleless vascular access systems when available. Place sharps in puncture-resistant containers.

Patient care equipment: Wear gloves if visibly contaminated. Handle equipment in a manner that prevents transfer of microorganisms to others and the environment. Clean, disinfect, and reprocess equipment before use with another patient. Pay special attention to frequently touched surfaces within the ambulance (e.g., handrails, seats, cabinets, doors). Perform hand hygiene.

Linens: Transport in a manner that prevents skin and mucous membrane exposure and avoids transfer of microorganisms to others and to the environment.

Respiratory hygiene/cough etiquette: Instruct symptomatic patients to cover mouth/nose when sneezing or coughing. Use tissues and dispose of them in no-touch receptacles. Perform hand hygiene after touching tissues. Place a surgical mask on patient. If a mask cannot be used, maintain separation (> 3 feet), if possible.

Patient resuscitation: Use mouthpiece, resuscitation bag, or other ventilation devices to prevent contact with mouth and oral secretions.

Sources: Centers for Disease Control and Prevention 2007. World Health Organization 2006.

Documentation

- Standard precautions used
- Personal protective equipment (PPE) used

Designated Infection Control Officer

The federal Ryan White Law, Subpart II, requires that every emergency response agency have a designated infection control officer (DICO). This individual is charged with ensuring that proper postexposure medical treatment and counseling are provided to the exposed employee/volunteer. Postexposure medical treatment is offered to prevent the exposed health care provider from contracting the disease to which he or she was exposed. Treatment should be offered within 24 to 48 hours following an exposure, with the actual time frame based on the diagnosis; exposure to bacterial meningitis, for example, would require treatment within 24 hours. The DICO tracks and follows the correct time frames, serves as a liaison between the exposed individual and the medical facility, ensures that confidentiality is maintained, and makes sure that documentation adheres to guidelines. This is important for workers' compensation issues and, in some states, presumption issues.

The communication network for exposure reporting involves three individuals: the exposed EMT/paramedic, the DICO, and the treating physician. If you feel you sustained an exposure, call your DICO directly. It is the DICO's job to make the initial determination as to whether an actual exposure occurred. Each department must have a reporting system that complies with the Ryan White Law and the OSHA-required Exposure Control Plan.

Patient Confidentiality and HIPAA

- Communication between you and the patient is confidential and generally cannot be disclosed without the patient's permission or a court order.
- The Health Insurance Portability and Accountability Act (HIPAA) considers all patient information that you obtain in the course of providing medical treatment to be protected health information (PHI). This includes all medical information, treatment provided, and any information that could be used to identify the patient.
- It is not acceptable for EMS patient care reports to sit in a public area or to be easily accessible. "War stories" told by medics may subject them to liability.

Patient information shall only be disclosed or released:

- If the patient, guardian, executor, or other legally authorized person has requested in writing that the information be released to a specific person, entity, or company.
- In compliance with a subpoena, judicial order, or applicable law, rule, and/or regulation.
- To process a claim for insurance, including Medicare or Medicaid, if authorized by the patient, guardian, executor, or other legally authorized person.
- To department staff in the performance of their duties and/or while conducting an inspection, audit, and/or investigation.
- To affect the transfer of the patient to another health care professional receiving the patient.

Documentation

- Patient consent to treatment and transport.

Social Media Tips (e.g., Facebook, Twitter)

1. Don't post inappropriate pictures or images, including any patient/provider identifiers.
2. Don't complain about your job, supervisors, or co-workers in a public forum.
3. Don't post inappropriate "statuses."
4. Be particular about your friends and associations.
5. Check your privacy and security settings and know their rules.
6. Consider establishing a "professional" profile page.
7. Don't use social networking while engaged in patient care or work activities.
8. Don't misrepresent yourself or others.
9. Be who you are.
10. Respect copyright and fair use laws.

Adapted from FireRescue1 News, *Don't Get Fired for Facebook: 10 Ways to Use Social Media Safely*, by Steve Wirth and Doug Wolfberg, July 28, 2010, http://www.firerescue1.com/print.asp?act=print&vid=859991.

Patient Refusal

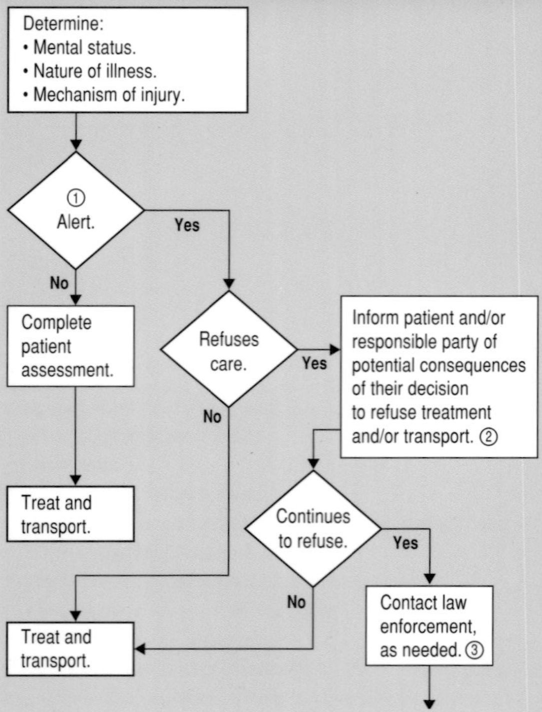

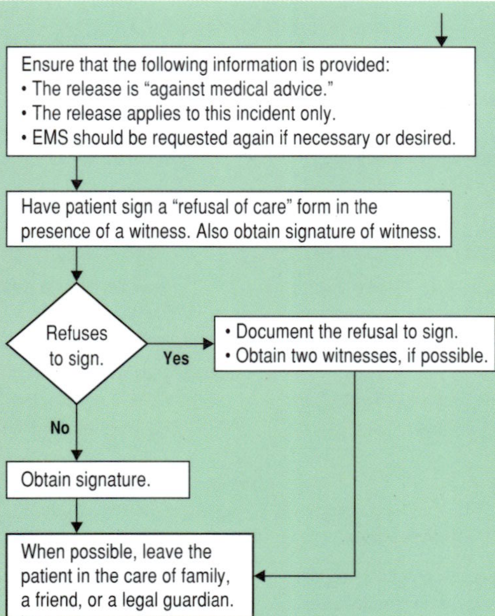

Note: This protocol assumes that it is medically indicated to treat or transport this patient.

1. "Alert" implies that the patient is conscious and oriented to person, place, and time.
2. Emancipated minor: An individual who is under the legal age but, because of other circumstances, is free from parental control and supervision via a court order.
3. EMS cannot forcibly restrain/transport a patient that is: alert, oriented, not a threat to themselves, or refusing medical treatment and/or transport.

Requesting an Air Medical Unit (AMU)

Considerations

Patients can be transported by ground or air. The goal is to get the patient to the emergency department safely in the least possible amount of time. Consider air transport if any one of the following situations are present:

TABLE 1 Guidelines to Request an On-scene Helicopter

Environmental Factors	Indicators of Severe Anatomic or Physiologic Compromise
• The time needed to transport a patient by ground to an appropriate facility poses a threat to the patient's survival and recovery.	• Unconsciousness or decreasing level of consciousness.
• Weather, road, and traffic conditions would seriously delay the patient's access to Advanced Life Support (ALS).	• Systolic blood pressure less than 90 mm Hg (adult trauma only).
• Critical care personnel and equipment are needed to adequately care for the patient during transport.	• Respiratory rate less than 10 per minute or greater than 30 per minute (adult trauma only).
• Falls of 20 feet or more.	• Glasgow Coma Scale score less than 10.
• Motor vehicle crashes (MVC) of **20 mph** or more without restraints.	• Compromised airway.
• Rearward displacement of front of car by **20 inches.**	• Penetrating injury to chest, abdomen, head, neck, or groin.
• Rearward displacement of front axle.	• Two or more femur or humerus fractures.
• Passenger compartment intrusion **18 inches** or greater.	• Flail chest.

Environmental Factors	Indicators of Severe Anatomic or Physiologic Compromise
• Ejection of patient from vehicle.	• Amputation proximal to wrist or ankle.
• Rollover	• Paralysis or spinal cord injury
• Deformity of a contact point (steering wheel, windshield, dashboard)	• Severe burns
• Death of occupant in the same vehicle	
• Pedestrian struck at **20 mph** or more	

Accessing the Air Medical Unit

The AMU is accessed through the New Jersey Regional Emergency Medical Communications System (REMCS) by calling **1-800-332-4356.** REMCS dispatches all air medical emergency services for all municipalities.

If your patient needs air transport, CALL FOR AN AMU NO MATTER WHAT TIME IT IS OR WHAT THE WEATHER CONDITIONS ARE!

Documentation

- Time of request
- Communication with REMCS

Requesting BLS/ALS

New Jersey 9-1-1 Dispatch

Emergency Medical Dispatchers will initiate either BLS dispatch or simultaneous ALS/BLS dispatch based on "State of New Jersey Emergency Medical Dispatch Guidecards." Criteria for ALS dispatch include, but are not limited to:

- Unconscious or not breathing normally
- Uncontrolled bleeding after attempts to control bleeding
- Vomiting blood or coffee-grounds material
- Burns over 20% of body surface area
- Femur fracture
- Falls greater than 10 feet
- Multiple casualty incidents
- Unusual behavior/acting strange
- Chest pain
- Respiratory distress
- Stroke
- New onset of altered mental status

Abdominal Pain, Nausea, and/or Vomiting

Considerations

- Allow patient to assume a position of comfort.
- Patient should not take anything by mouth.
- Abdominal pain may be cardiac in origin, especially in older women.

Assessment

- Airway, breathing, circulation.
- Administer oxygen, as needed.
- Obtain history.
- Look for medical alert tags, signs of overdose, and trauma.
- Ask the following:
  - Have there been previous episodes?
  - When was the patient's last meal?
  - What are the patient's current medications?
  - If female, when was the patient's last menstrual period?
  - Is it possible that the patient is pregnant?
- Abdominal exam: Note pain (nature, duration, intensity, radiation on 1–10 scale). Note associated signs and symptoms (nausea, vomiting, bowel tones, guarding, rebound tenderness, distention).

Treatment

- ABCs.
- Oxygen, as needed, SpO_2.
- Obtain history. ①

↓

Abdominal exam. ②

↓

Allow patient to assume position of comfort.

↓

NPO: Nothing by mouth.

↓

Nausea, vomiting. ③

↓

Transport.

1. Ischemic cardiac pain can present as abdominal pain, especially in older female patients.
2. Note pain (nature, duration, intensity, radiation on 1–10 scale). Auscultate prior to palpation. Observe for palpable mass; avoid palpation if you suspect an abdominal mass. Note associated signs and symptoms (nausea, vomiting, bowel tones, guarding, rebound tenderness, distention).
3. Consider ALS for severe nausea/vomiting. ALS may administer Ondansetron hydrochloride (Zofran) 4 mg IV over 2 minutes. May repeat in 10 minutes if symptoms not resolved. Ondansetron hydrochloride (Zofran) should be used with caution in patients with impaired liver function. Ondansetron hydrochloride (Zofran) does not prevent motion sickness and is not recommended for children younger than 12 years.

Documentation

- Signs and symptoms
- Cardiac rhythm, if obtained
- Nature, intensity, and duration of pain
- Vital signs
- Oxygen saturation (SpO_2)
- Treatment
- Response to treatment

Abuse and Neglect

Considerations

Abuse takes many forms, and some people suffer from more than one kind of abuse.

- Abuse is the physical, sexual, or emotional harm or risk of harm to another, such as a child, elder, or spouse.
- Child abuse is the physical, sexual, or emotional harm or risk of harm to a child under the age of 18.
- Neglect occurs when a parent or caregiver fails to provide proper supervision or adequate food, clothing, shelter, education, or medical care although financially able or assisted to do so.

Physical Abuse

Physical signs: Bruises, welts, cuts, scars, broken bones, burns, other injuries, often in various stages of healing.

Behavioral signs: Wears clothing inappropriate for weather to hide injuries, appears withdrawn or depressed, afraid or reluctant to go home, will shy away from physical contact, may be aggressive.

Sexual Abuse

Physical signs: Torn, stained, or bloody underwear; trouble walking or standing; pain, itching, bruises, or bleeding in the genital area; a sexually transmitted disease.

Behavioral signs: Has an unusual knowledge of sex or acts seductively, fear of a particular person, withdrawal or depression, sudden weight gain or loss, shies away from physical contact, runs away from home.

Emotional Abuse

Physical signs: Speech disorders, slow physical development.

Behavioral signs: Acts too mature or too childish for his or her age, has difficulty making and/or keeping friends, extreme behavioral changes.

Neglect

Physical signs: Poor hygiene, slow physical development, or may appear underweight; unattended medical needs; little or no supervision at home.

Behavioral signs: Arrives at school or work very early or late or misses school or work often, frequently tired or hungry, steals food, dresses inappropriately for the weather.

If You Suspect Abuse

- Watch for signs
- Be approachable
- Evaluate the situation
- Report it

If Someone Tells You About Abuse

- Be a good listener
- Be supportive
- Don't overreact
- Write it down and report it

Reporting Abuse or Neglect

Children

If you suspect child abuse, or a child tells you about abuse, don't delay. You must report it! Everyone in New Jersey is required to report suspected abuse. To make a report, call the NJ Division of Youth and Family Services' toll-free Child Abuse Hotline 24 hours a day, 7 days a week: 1-877-NJ-ABUSE (1-877-652-2873) TTY 1-800-835-5510.

Adults

If you or someone you know is 18 years of age or older; living in the community; and is subject to abuse, neglect, and/or exploitation; a county Adult Protective Services (APS) program may be the place to turn! There is an APS program in each of the 21 counties that is monitored and evaluated by state staff. Complainants may be clients, caregivers, family members, agencies, or any interested or involved individuals. Calls may be made to the particular county APS office or to the Public Awareness, Information, Assistance, and Outreach Unit at 1-800-792-8820.

Elders

The Office of the Ombudsman for the Institutionalized Elderly investigates and responds to complaints of abuse, neglect, and exploitation of individuals 60 years of age and older who reside in licensed facilities within New Jersey, both public and private. To make a report, call 1-877-582-6995.

County Adult Protective Services (APS) Offices

Atlantic
Atlantic County Division of Intergenerational Services
Phone: 1-888-426-9243

Bergen
Bergen County Board of Social Services
Phone: 201-368-4300
After hours: 1-800-624-0275

Burlington
Burlington County Board of Social Services
Phone: 609-261-1000
After hours: 1-866-234-5006 or 856-234-8888

Camden
Camden County Board of Social Services
Phone: 856-225-8178

Cape May
Cape May County Board of Social Services
Phone: 609-886-6200

Cumberland
Cumberland County Guidance Center
Phone: 856-825-6810 Ext. 299

Essex
FOCUS, Hispanic Center for Human Dev., Inc.
Phone: 973-624-2528 Ext. 135 or 1-866-90-FOCUS

Gloucester
Gloucester County Board of Social Services
Phone: 856-582-9200 or 856-256-2150

Hudson
Hudson County Protective Services, Inc.
Phone: 201-295-5160

Hunterdon
Hunterdon County Department of Human Services
Phone: 908-788-1300
After hours: 908-782-HELP or 908-735-HELP

Mercer
Mercer County Board of Social Services
Phone: 609-989-4346 or 609-989-4347

Middlesex
Middlesex County Board of Social Services
Phone: 732-745-3635

Monmouth
Family and Children Services of Monmouth County
Phone: 732-531-9191
After hours: 732-222-9111 or 1-800-495-0005

Morris
Morris County Aging, Disabilities and Veterans
Phone: 973-326-7282, 973-326-7283
After hours: 973-285-2900

Ocean
Ocean County Board of Social Services
Phone: 732-349-1500
After hours: 732-240-6100

Passaic
Passaic County Board of Social Services
Phone: 973-881-2616
After hours: 973-345-2676

Salem
Salem County Office on Aging
Phone: 856-935-7510 Ext. 8622 or 856-339-8622

Somerset
Somerset County Board of Social Services
Phone: 908-526-8800
After hours: 1-800-287-3607

Sussex
Sussex County Division of Social Services
Phone: 973-383-3600
After hours: 1-800-446-6963

Union
Catholic Community Services
Phone: 908-497-3902

Warren
Warren County Division of Senior Services
Phone: 908-475-6591

What to Report

Report the person's name, age, and address. Report the name of the suspected abuser and his or her relationship with the person. Report the type of abuse suspected, any knowledge of past abuse, whether there are witnesses, and your relationship to the person. If you do not have all this information, it is still your responsibility to make a report.

Hives, itching, normal perfusion, no dyspnea.

Diphenhydramine (Benadryl) 50 mg.

Observe closely.

Moderate reaction.

Dyspnea, wheeze, edema, hives, normal perfusion.

Establish vascular access.

Diphenhydramine (Benadryl) 50 mg.

Severe reaction.

Consider epinephrine
BLS: Auto-injector. (1)
ALS: Epinephrine 1:1,000 0.3 mL IM. (2)

Severe dyspnea, wheeze, poor perfusion, edema.

Administer fluid bolus. (3)

Diphenhydramine (Benadryl) (4) 50–100 mg.

continues

Treatment, continued

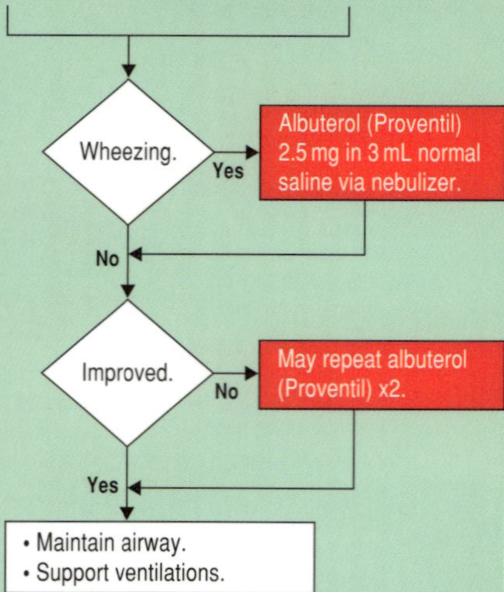

1. If your BLS agency is a NJDHSS registered epinephrine auto-injector agency, follow NJDHSS written protocol (www.state.nj.us/health/ems). If your BLS agency is not a DHSS registered epinephrine auto-injector agency, you can only assist the patient in using his or her own epinephrine auto-injector as needed.
2. Epinephrine: Use ONLY if the patient is hypotensive or in severe respiratory distress. Use cautiously in patients over 45 years of age. May repeat if there is no improvement noted 5 minutes after the initial administration.
3. Normal Saline: Administer IV fluid bolus if the patient is hypotensive. Repeat once if systolic blood pressure remains below 100 mm Hg.
4. Diphenhydramine may be given IM if IV access is delayed or not available. IV rate of administration: 50 mg over 2 minutes.

Pediatric Considerations

BLS

- If under age 4, consider pediatric epinephrine auto-injector.
- Consider medical command.

ALS

- Epinephrine: 1:1,000: 0.01 mg/kg (0.01 mL/kg) IM (max 0.3 mg).
- Albuterol (Proventil): 2.5 mg in 3 mL NS via nebulizer, if wheezing is present.
- Establish vascular access.
- If hypotensive, administer IV NS 20 mL/kg.
- If no improvement, administer diphenhydramine hydrochloride (Benadryl) 1 mg/kg IV/IO to a maximum of 50 mg slowly (over 2 minutes).
- Contact medical command.

Documentation

- Respiratory effort/quality
- Glasgow Coma Scale (GCS) score
- Skin color
- Capillary refill
- Response to treatment

Altered Mental Status

Considerations

Possible causes: Head injury, diabetes, overdose, cardiac or respiratory arrest, arrhythmias, seizure, hypertension, hypotension, stoke.

- Consider *Stroke and Cerebrovascular Accidents* protocol.
- Consider *Diabetic Emergencies* protocol.

Assessment

- Airway, breathing, circulation.
- Administer 100% oxygen.
- Assist ventilations via bag-valve mask (BVM), as needed.
- BLS to request ALS.
- Transport ASAP.
- Look for medical alert tags, signs of overdose, trauma. Bring medication bottles to ED.
- Keep patient warm.

Treatment

- ABCs.
- Oxygen 100%, SpO_2.
- Assist ventilations, as needed.

↓

- Cardiac monitor.
- Establish vascular access.
- Check blood glucose.

↓

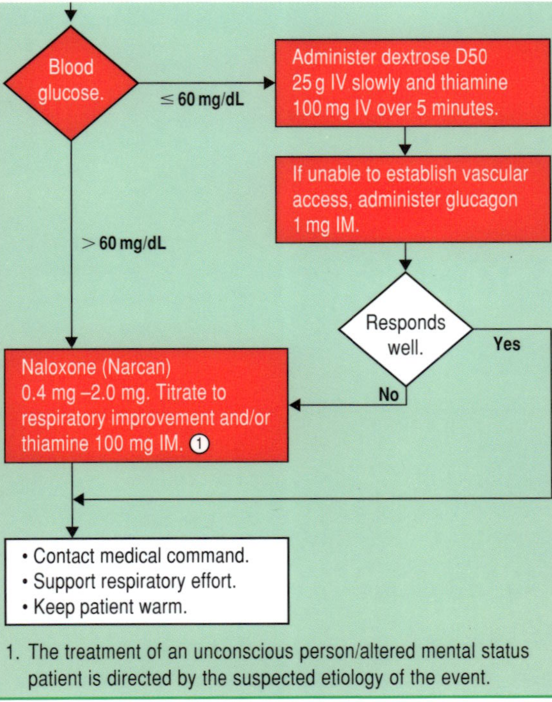

1. The treatment of an unconscious person/altered mental status patient is directed by the suspected etiology of the event.

Pediatric Considerations

ALS

- Dextrose: Patients younger than 1 month, administer dextrose 10% solution, D10, 0.5 g/kg slow IV/IO; patients 1 month or older, administer dextrose 25% solution, D25, 0.5 g/kg slow IV/IO.
- If unable to establish vascular access, administer glucagon 0.1 mg/kg IM, to a maximum of 1 mg. (1 mg = 1 mL = 1 unit).
- If there is no change in the patient's mental status and there are signs of possible opioid toxicity, administer naloxone hydrochloride (Narcan) 0.2 mg.
- If no responses, administer naloxone hydrochloride (Narcan) 0.1 mg/kg to a maximum of 2 mg.
- If there is a history of dehydration, and vascular access has been established administer fluid bolus NS 20 mL/kg.
- Contact medical command.

Documentation

- Glasgow Coma Scale (GCS) score
- Clinical response to medications
- Blood glucose level
- Oxygen saturation (SpO_2)
- Total IV fluids
- Medical history
- Vital signs
- Cardiac rhythm

Behavioral Emergencies and Psychiatric Disorders

Considerations

- Ensure your personal safety.
- Request law enforcement, as needed.
- Approach the patient only when it is safe to do so. Speak in an even, reassuring manner.

Assessment

- Airway, breathing, circulation.
- Administer oxygen, as needed.
- Obtain history (consider possibility of hypoglycemia).
- Look for medic alert tags.
- Is the patient a danger to self or others? Request that law enforcement assist with transport.
- Is the patient suicidal? Do not leave patient alone. Remove any dangerous objects.
- Is the patient alert? If not alert, provide oxygen. See *Altered Mental Status* protocol.
- Is the patient agitated? Consider your own safety and request law enforcement assistance, as needed.
- Is the patient violent? Restrain in lateral recumbent position or supine.
- Transport to the most appropriate facility.

Treatment

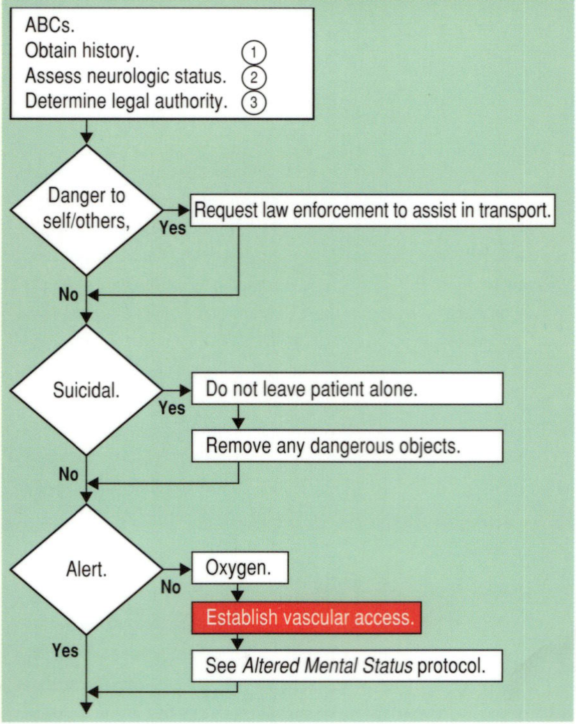
ABCs.
Obtain history. ①
Assess neurologic status. ②
Determine legal authority. ③
Danger to self/others,
Yes
Request law enforcement to assist in transport.
No
Suicidal.
Yes
Do not leave patient alone.
Remove any dangerous objects.
No
Alert.
No
Oxygen.
Establish vascular access.
See *Altered Mental Status* protocol.
Yes

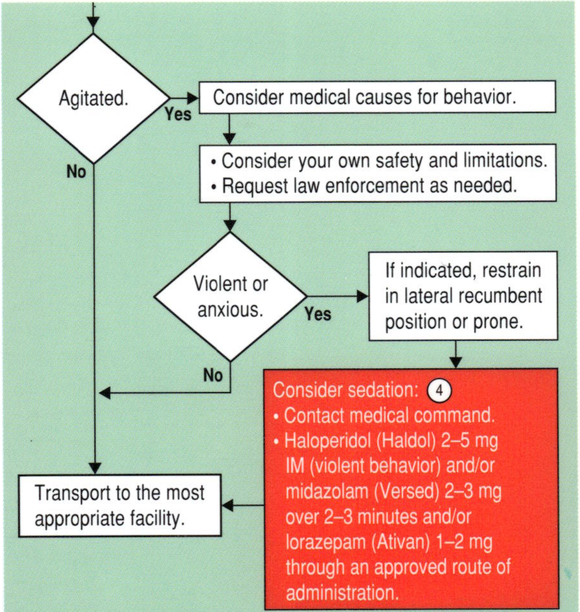

1. Note bizarre behavior, abrupt change in behavior, suicidal ideation, possible drug or alcohol ingestion, history of diabetes, etc. Look for medic alert tag.
2. Consider the possibility of hypoglycemia. Low blood glucose can cause agitation, confusion, and irritability.

continues

Treatment, continued

3. Do you have the legal authority and responsibility to provide care? Consult with law enforcement and medical command if you have any questions.
4. Use caution for patients presenting with a fever.

Documentation

- Behavior
- Speech patterns
- Suicidal ideation
- Glasgow Coma Scale (GCS) score
- Level of cooperation
- Skin color
- Medical history
- Current medications
- Communication with law enforcement
- Contact with medical command or other authorities

Diabetic Emergencies

Assessment

- Airway, breathing, circulation.
- Administer 100% oxygen via nonrebreathing mask, as needed; assist ventilations, as needed.
- Perform physical examination.
- Keep patient warm.
- Transport.
- BLS to consider ALS.

Treatment

- ABCs.
- Oxygen 100% via NRB mask, SpO_2.
- Assist ventilations, as needed.

↓

Cardiac monitor.

↓

If airway patent, gag reflex present, with ability to swallow, administer oral glucose.

↓

continues

Treatment, continued

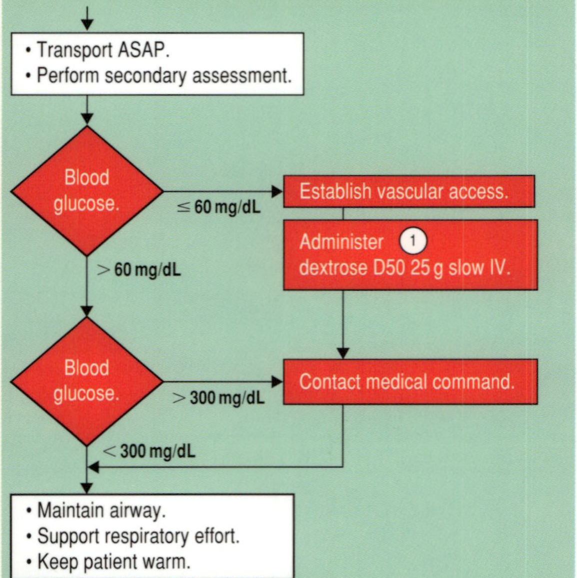

1. If unable to start IV for dextrose, administer glucagon 1 mg IM.

Pediatric Considerations

ALS

Dextrose: Patients younger than 1 month, administer dextrose 10% solution D10, 0.5 g/kg slow IV/IO; patients 1 month or older administer dextrose 25% solution D25, 0.5 g/kg slow IV/IO.

If unable to establish vascular access for dextrose, may give children older than 8 years glucagon 0.1 mg/kg up to 1 mg IM.

Documentation

- Respiratory effort
- Oxygen saturation (SpO_2)
- Blood glucose level
- IV fluid totals
- Response to dextrose
- Skin color
- Glasgow Coma Scale (GCS) score
- Cardiac rhythm

Frostbite

Assessment

- Airway, breathing, circulation.
- Administer 100% oxygen.
- Check core temperature. If the patient's temperature is < 95°F (35°C), see the *Hypothermia* protocol.
- Protect affected area from friction, pressure, and trauma.
- Do not allow the patient to ambulate.
- Keep the patient warm.
- Provide warm fluids orally if the patient's gag reflex is intact.
- Apply oxygen saturation (SpO_2) probe to detect peripheral perfusion.
- Transport.

Treatment

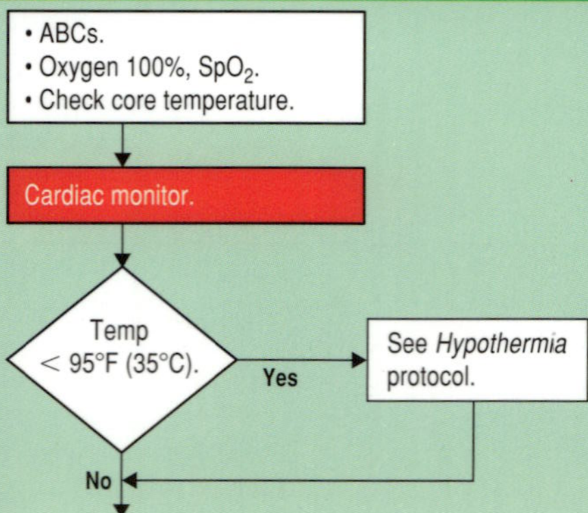

- Focus assessment on injured areas.
- Protect areas from friction, pressure, trauma.
- Do not allow patient to ambulate.
- Keep patient warm.
- May give warm fluids orally if gag reflex intact.

↓

Apply SpO_2 probe to a non-affected digit to detect peripheral perfusion.

↓

Consider medication to control pain.

↓

Transport.

Documentation

- Signs and symptoms
- Oxygen saturation (SpO_2)
- Glasgow Coma Scale (GCS) score
- Cardiac rhythm
- Core temperature
- Mechanism of injury/exposure
- Treatment
- Response to treatment

Hypoperfusion: Nontraumatic Shock

Considerations (Adult Patient)

- Signs and symptoms of shock include a pulse > 120 beats/min, systolic blood pressure < 90 mm Hg, delayed capillary refill, confusion, restlessness, apathy, postural hypotension/syncope, cool/moist skin.

Assessment

- Airway, breathing, circulation.
- Administer 100% oxygen. Assist ventilations, as needed.
- Transport ASAP.
- BLS to consider ALS (IV fluids, advanced airway).
- Calculate Glasgow Coma Scale (GCS) score.

Treatment

(1)
- ABCs.
- Oxygen 100%, SpO_2.
- Assist ventilations, as needed.

↓

- Cardiac monitor.
- Establish vascular access.
- Administer fluid bolus.

↓

- Reassess vital signs and condition of the patient.
- Contact medical command.

↓

- Keep patient warm.
- Transport and notify receiving hospital ASAP.
- Monitor respiratory status/SpO_2.
- ALS: Monitor cardiac rhythm.

This protocol is authorized in the event that an adult presents with significant and symptomatic hypotension (systolic BP < 90 mm Hg) unaccompanied by bradycardia or trauma, with patient exhibiting signs of shock due to dehydration, sepsis, and nontraumatic hemorrhage (i.e., GI bleeding).

1. Septic shock is a medical emergency. Expedite transport! Suspect sepsis in patients who have an infection and/or have at least two of the following: temperature > 100.4°F (38°C) or < 96.8°F (36°C), respiratory rate of > 32 breaths/min, or pulse > 90 beats/min. Advise the receiving facility that you suspect sepsis.

Pediatric Considerations

BLS

- Maintain normal body temperature.
- Contact medical command.

ALS

- Maintain normal body temperature.
- Establish vascular access.
- Administer NS 20 mL/kg IV.
- Check blood glucose. If blood glucose < 60 mg/dL: For patients younger than 1 month of age, administer 0.5 g/kg of a D10 solution IV/IO; for patients older than 1 month of age, administer 0.5 g/kg of a D25 solution IV/IO.
  - If unable to establish IV/IO, administer glucagon 0.1 mg/kg to a maximum of 1 mg via IM.
- If no change, repeat IV NS bolus.
- Contact medical command.

Documentation

- Respiratory effort
- Oxygen saturation (SpO_2)
- Cardiac rhythm
- Capillary refill
- GCS score
- Lung sounds
- Quality of pulses
- Skin color, temperature, and moisture

Hyperthermia

Considerations

- Prevent patient from shivering.

Assessment

- Airway, breathing, circulation.
- Administer 100% oxygen.
- Transport ASAP.
- Cooling measures:
  - Move patient to a cool environment (shade, air conditioning).
  - Fan patient.
  - Apply moist dressings.
  - Give cool fluids orally if gag reflex is intact.

Treatment

- ABCs.
- Oxygen 100%, SpO_2.
- Assist ventilations, as needed.
- Move patient to a cool environment.
- Take temperature and assess vital signs.

↓

Cardiac monitor.

↓

continues

Treatment, continued

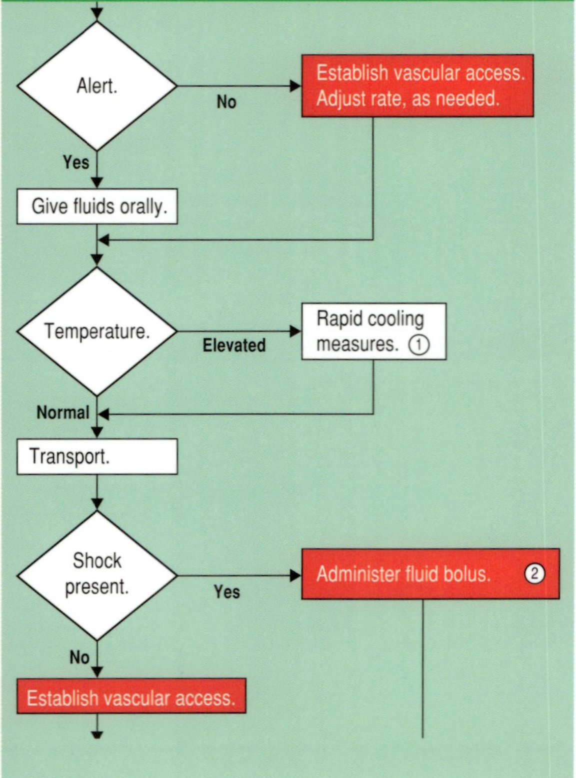

Monitor:

- ALS: Monitor cardiac rhythm.
- Vital signs.
- LOC, SpO_2.
- Anticipate potential seizure activity.

1. Move patient to a cool environment. Fan patient, apply moist dressings, prevent shivering.
2. Monitor patient response to IV fluids closely. Blood pressure will usually return to normal quickly. Administer IV fluids, as needed. Do not overload the patient.

Documentation

- Signs and symptoms
- Oxygen saturation (SpO_2)
- Glasgow Coma Scale (GCS) score
- Cardiac rhythm
- Core temperature
- Mechanism of injury/exposure
- Treatment
- Response to treatment

Hypothermia

Considerations

- Remove wet clothing.
- Prevent heat loss/wind chill.
- Avoid rough movement.

Assessment

- Airway, breathing, circulation.
- Administer oxygen, as needed.
- Perform CPR, as needed.
- Maintain horizontal position.
- Monitor core temperature.
  - **Mild hypothermia**: 93°–96.8°F (34°–36°C)—passive rewarming needed.
  - **Moderate hypothermia**: 86°–93°F (30°–34°C)—active external rewarming needed.
  - **Severe hypothermia**: < 86°F (30°C)—active internal warming needed.
- AED, as needed.
- BLS to consider ALS.
- Transport ASAP.
- Warming methods include warm water bottles, heating pads, radiant heat sources, and warming beds. Apply hot packs and/or hot water bottles to axilla and groin. Do not burn the patient. Keep the ambulance's patient care area warm.

Treatment

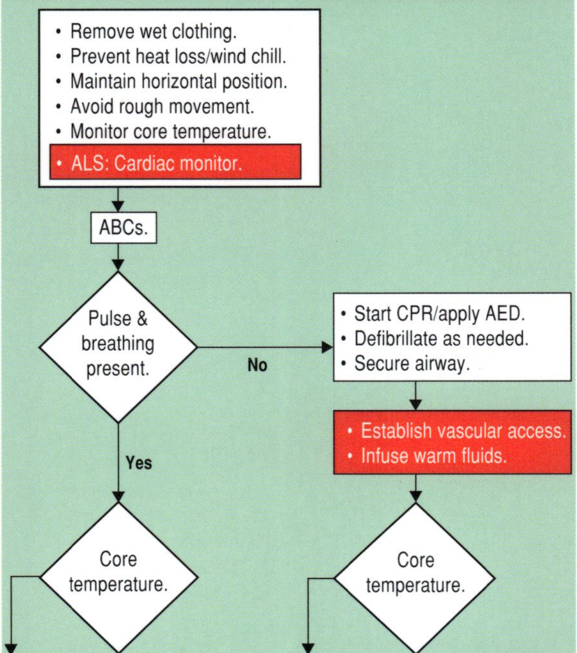

continues

Treatment, continued

93° – 96.8°F (34 – 36°C):
Mild hypothermia
- Passive rewarming needed.

86° – 93°F (30 – 34°C): ①
Moderate hypothermia
- Active external rewarming of truncal areas needed.

< 86°F (30°C):
Severe hypothermia
- Active internal warming needed.

< 86°F (30°C)
- Continue CPR.
- ALS: Withhold IV meds.
- Transport ASAP.

> 86°F (30°C) ②
- Continue CPR.
- ALS: Give IV meds as needed.
- Defibrillate as needed.

Active internal rewarming.
- Warm IV fluid.

Continue internal rewarming until:
- Core temperature > 95°F (35°C), or
- Return of spontaneous circulation, or
- Resuscitative measures cease.

- Notify receiving hospital ASAP.
- ALS: Monitor cardiac rhythm.
- Monitor core temperature, vital signs, SpO_2.
- Transport ASAP.

1. Warming methods include warm water bottles, hot packs, and blankets. Apply hot packs and/or hot water bottles to axilla and groin. Do not burn the patient. Keep the ambulance's patient care area warm.
2. Give IV medications at longer than standard intervals.

Documentation

- Signs and symptoms
- Oxygen saturation (SpO_2)
- Cardiac rhythm
- Core temperature
- Mechanism of injury/exposure
- Treatment
- Response to treatment

Near Drowning

Considerations

- The rescue from the water should be performed by a trained rescuer with the appropriate equipment and support.
- Aggressive respiratory management is the key to effective treatment in drowning and near-drowning cases.

Assessment

- Remove the victim from the water.
- Airway, breathing, circulation.
- Protect c-spine if fall or diving accident suspected.
- Administer 100% oxygen. While patient is being rescued, assist ventilations, as needed.
- BLS to consider ALS.
- Keep patient warm. Remove wet clothing. Apply hot packs if the patient is cold.
- Transport ASAP. All near-drowning victims should be examined by a physician.

Treatment

- Remove victim from water. (1)
- Airway. (2)
- Transport ASAP. (3)

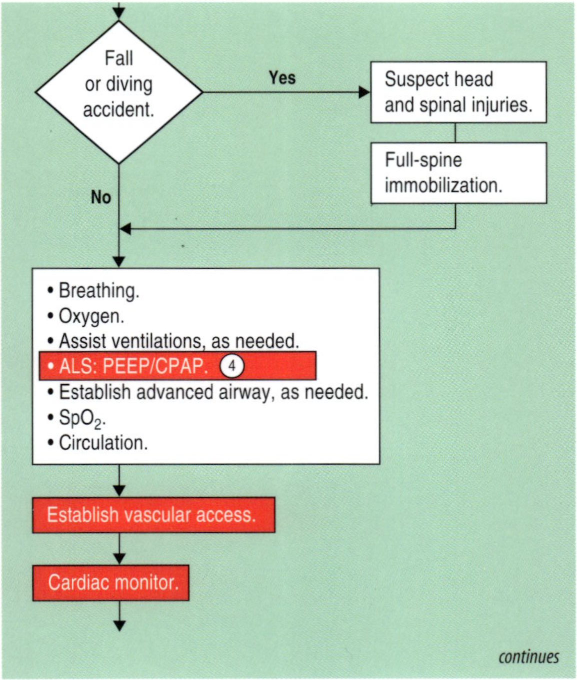
Fall or diving accident.
Yes
Suspect head and spinal injuries.
Full-spine immobilization.
No
• Breathing.
• Oxygen.
• Assist ventilations, as needed.
• ALS: PEEP/CPAP. 4
• Establish advanced airway, as needed.
• SpO_2.
• Circulation.
Establish vascular access.
Cardiac monitor.

continues

Treatment, continued

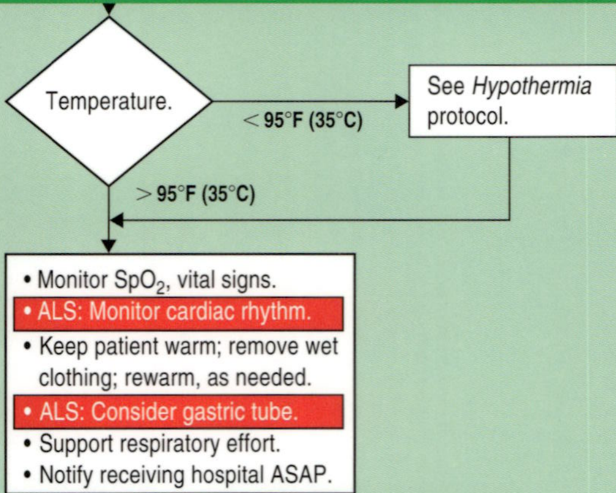

1. To be performed by a trained rescuer with appropriate equipment.
2. Ventilation should be initiated while the patient is being rescued.
3. All near-drowning victims should be examined by a physician.
4. Use a PEEP (positive end-expiratory pressure)/CPAP (continuous positive airway pressure) valve, if available.

Documentation

- Onset and duration of incident
- Respiratory effort
- Oxygen saturation (SpO_2)
- IV fluid totals
- Treatment
- Response to treatment
- Skin color
- Glasgow Coma Scale (GCS) score
- Cardiac rhythm
- Capillary refill

Pain Management

Considerations

- See the *Chest Pain* protocol if chest pain exists.
- Use the *Wong-Baker Faces Scale* to quantify the patient's pain level.

Assessment

- Airway, breathing, circulation.
- Administer oxygen, as needed.
- Assess pain level.
- BLS to consider ALS.
- Immobilize fractures/dislocations; elevate and apply ice, if appropriate.

Treatment

- ABCs.
- Oxygen, as needed, SpO_2.

↓

Cardiac monitor.

↓

Assess pain level:
Ask the patient to quantify pain on an analog pain scale (0 = no pain, 10 = most severe).

↓

continues

Treatment, continued

If fractures or dislocations exist, immobilize the extremity per protocol and elevate and apply ice if appropriate.

↓

For burn/trauma patients only:
Morphine 0.1 mg/kg up to 10 mg.
OR
Fentanyl 1 mcg/kg up to 100 mcg.
Titrate slowly.

↓

Contact medical command.

↓

- Monitor respiratory effort, LOC closely.
- Keep the patient warm.

Pediatric Considerations

ALS

Morphine and fentanyl dosages are identical for both pediatric and adult patients.

Documentation

- Dose
- Pain level
- Complications or absence of complications of medication administration
- Effectiveness
- Respiratory effort

Seizures

Considerations

- Seizures in children should be taken seriously. Febrile seizures usually last no longer than 5 minutes and resolve without medications. Consider cooling measures.
- Causes of seizures include overdose, epilepsy, and cerebral neoplasm.
- Provide a quiet, reassuring environment during transport.

Assessment

- Airway, breathing, circulation.
- Administer oxygen if respiratory effort or rate is abnormal.
- BLS to request ALS.
- Look for medical alert tags, signs of overdose, trauma.
- Transport ASAP.
- Anticipate additional seizures.

Treatment

- ABCs.
- Administer oxygen if respiratory effort or rate are abnormal or SpO_2 is below 95%.

↓

- Protect patient from injury during and after seizure.
- Place in lateral recumbent position if trauma is absent.
- Obtain vital signs.

↓

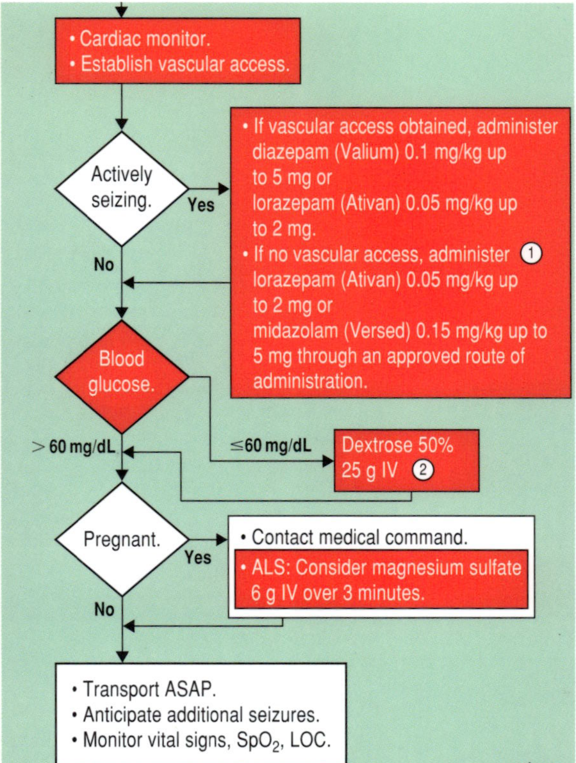
• Cardiac monitor.
• Establish vascular access.
Actively seizing.
Yes
• If vascular access obtained, administer diazepam (Valium) 0.1 mg/kg up to 5 mg or lorazepam (Ativan) 0.05 mg/kg up to 2 mg.
• If no vascular access, administer ① lorazepam (Ativan) 0.05 mg/kg up to 2 mg or midazolam (Versed) 0.15 mg/kg up to 5 mg through an approved route of administration.
No
Blood glucose.
$>$ 60 mg/dL
$\leq$60 mg/dL
Dextrose 50% 25 g IV ②
Pregnant.
Yes
• Contact medical command.
• ALS: Consider magnesium sulfate 6 g IV over 3 minutes.
No
• Transport ASAP.
• Anticipate additional seizures.
• Monitor vital signs, SpO_2, LOC.

continues

Treatment, continued

1. Consider lorazepam (Ativan): Administer IV diluted 1:1 with normal saline.
2. Administer thiamine 100 mg prior to dextrose if you suspect alcoholism or malnutrition.

Pediatric Considerations

ALS

- Diazapam (Valium): May be administered rectally if vascular access route is not available. To administer rectally, draw the appropriate IV dose into a tuberculosis syringe, remove the needle, and gently insert the syringe into the patient's rectum.
- Valium, Ativan, and Versed dosages are identical for both pediatric and adult patients.

Documentation

- Glasgow Coma Scale (GCS) score
- Clinical response to medications
- Blood glucose level
- Oxygen saturation (SpO_2)
- Total IV fluids administered
- Medical history
- Cardiac rhythm
- Physical activity during/before seizure
- Length of seizure

Stroke and Cerebrovascular Accidents

Considerations

- Stroke treatment is time sensitive. If the signs and symptoms of stroke have been identified, transport should be initiated without delay and the receiving hospital notified.
- If the patient is hemodynamically stable and/or without airway compromise, they should be transported to the closest New Jersey-designated stroke center.
- If the patient is unstable (respiratory or hemodynamically) and is accompanied by BLS only, then the patient is to be transported to the closest, most appropriate hospital regardless of stroke center status.

Assessment

- Airway, breathing, circulation.
- Administer oxygen, as needed.
- Perform the ACT F.A.S.T. stroke assessment, Cincinnati Prehospital Stroke Scale assessment, or Los Angeles Prehospital Stroke Screen.
- BLS to call for ALS but not delay transport awaiting their arrival.
- Determine time of onset, which is defined as the last time the patient was seen or spoken to in a normal state. If possible, obtain the name and cell phone number of the witness and provide this to the receiving facility.
- Patients who are stable should be transported to a designated stroke center with notification to receiving facility.
- Perform a detailed neurologic assessment. Calculate Glascow Coma Scale (GCS) score.

Treatment

- ABCs.
- Oxygen, SpO_2.
- Transport ASAP. (1)

↓

- Monitor cardiac rhythm.
- Obtain 12-Lead ECG.
- Establish vascular access. (2)

↓

Blood glucose.

$\le$ 60 mg/dL → Dextrose 50% 25 g IV. → Advise receiving facility ASAP

$>$ 60 mg/dL ↓

Advise receiving facility ASAP of time of onset, signs/symptoms. (3)

↓

Prepare to suction airway, as needed.

↓

Contact medical command.

↓

Do NOT treat hypertension in the field.

1. Do NOT delay transport at any time in this protocol. Patients with acute stroke signs and symptoms should be transported to a designated stroke center.
2. Glucose-containing solutions should be avoided unless hypoglycemia is documented by a rapid glucose test.
3. If possible, obtain the name and cell phone number of a witness and provide this to the receiving facility.

Documentation

- Time of onset
- Duration of incident
- Results of detailed neurologic assessment
- GCS score
- Respiratory effort
- Oxygen saturation (SpO_2)
- Cardiac rhythm
- Capillary refill

Chest Pain and Acute Myocardial Infarction

Considerations

- Contact medical command any time you have concerns or questions.

Assessment

- Airway, breathing, circulation.
- Oxygen 100%.
- BLS to request ALS.
- Place the patient in a position of comfort.
- **BLS: Nitroglycerin administration:** You may assist the patient to administer nitroglycerin 0.4 mg if:
  - The patient possesses his or her own prescribed nitroglycerin in either tablet or spray form (0.4 mg per dose),
  - AND the patient's systolic blood pressure is equal to or greater than 100 mm Hg,
  - AND the patient has NOT taken the maximum of three doses within the past 15 minutes.
- Nitroglycerin is contraindicated if the patient is taking Viagra, Levitra, Cialis, or another erectile dysfunction medication.
- Monitor relief of discomfort after interventions using a pain scale of 1 to 10.
- **BLS: Aspirin administration:** You may assist the patient with the administration of aspirin up to 325 mg if:
  - The patient is at least 19 years old
  - AND the patient has NOT taken the maximum 325 mg dose for this episode

*Have patient chew then swallow the aspirin (even if not a "chewable" tablet).

Procedure for Nitroglycerin Administration

1. Check the medication's expiration date. Do not administer if expired.
2. Assist in the administration of one tablet or spray under the patient's tongue.
3. Wait 2 minutes before reassessing the patient's chest pain or chest discomfort. Reassess vital signs.

- If the chest pain continues AND the systolic blood pressure remains > 100 mm Hg, you may repeat the administration of one dose.
- You may give up to three doses within a 10–15 minute time frame, provided the patient has not already taken one or more doses during the time frame. If pain free for more than 15 minutes and pain returns, this is considered a new onset. May administer an additional three doses.

Contraindications to Nitroglycerin Administration

- Hypotension (a systolic blood pressure < 100 mm Hg)
- Recent head injury
- Infants and children
- Patients who have already taken three doses within the 15 minutes prior to your arrival
- Use of erectile dysfunction medications within the previous 72 hours

Contraindications to Aspirin Administration

- Known hypersensitivity or allergy to aspirin
- Bleeding or active bleeding disorder
- Third trimester pregnancy
- Abdominal pain or pulsations, suspicion of thoracic or abdominal aortic aneurysm
- The aspirin is expired
- Dosage taken prior to arrival

BLS Treatment

- ABCs.
- Oxygen, SpO_2. ①
- Vital signs.

↓

- Obtain medical history. ②
- Transport ASAP.

↓

continues

BLS Treatment, continued

↓

Assist/administer aspirin.

↓

Assist patient with nitroglycerin.
See Assessment section for guidelines.

1. Oxygen: Adjust flow rate and route of administration, as needed. Consider hypoxic drive in COPD and degree of respiratory effort. Non-COPD patients should be able to maintain oxygen saturation (SpO_2) of 97% or higher. Increase oxygen concentration if SpO_2 is low.
2. History: Signs/symptoms; pain presentation, including location of pain, duration, onset, quality, relation to physical effort; history of coronary artery disease; use of aspirin and/or nitroglycerin; and use of erectile dysfunction medications.

ALS Treatment

- ABCs.
- Oxygen, SpO_2. ①
- Monitor cardiac rhythm.
- Vital signs.

↓

- Nitroglycerin SL 0.4 mg ② every 5 min, up to 1.2 mg. Repeat as needed for pain.
- Attempt vascular access; do not delay transport.

Acute myocardial infarction 12-lead EKG interpretation

Anterior wall:
- ST elevation in leads V1–V4

Inferior wall:
- ST elevation in leads II, III, aVF

Lateral wall:
- ST elevation in leads I, aVL, V5–V6

Posterior wall:
- ST depression and tall, broad (> 0.04 sec) R wave in leads V1 and V2 (reciprocal changes)

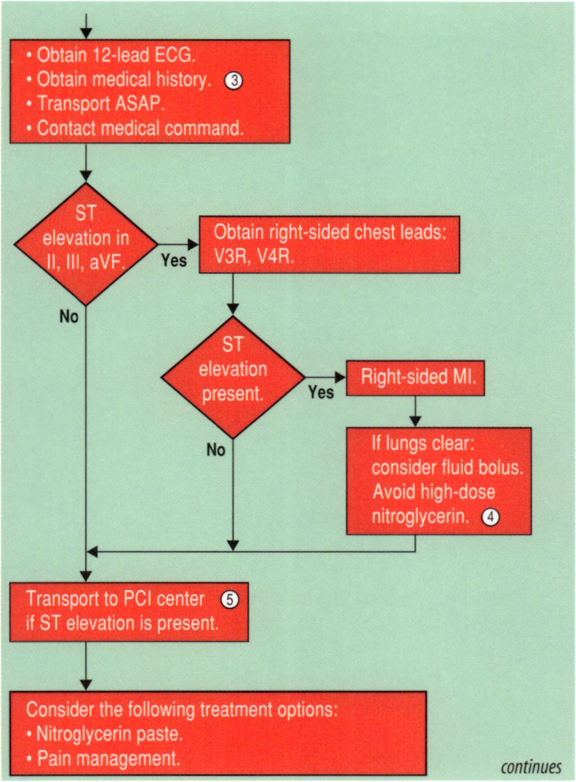
• Obtain 12-lead ECG.
• Obtain medical history. ③
• Transport ASAP.
• Contact medical command.
ST elevation in II, III, aVF.
Yes
No
Obtain right-sided chest leads: V3R, V4R.
ST elevation present.
Yes
No
Right-sided MI.
If lungs clear: consider fluid bolus. Avoid high-dose nitroglycerin. ④
Transport to PCI center ⑤ if ST elevation is present.
Consider the following treatment options:
• Nitroglycerin paste.
• Pain management.

continues

ALS Treatment, continued

1. Oxygen: Adjust flow rate and route of administration, as needed. Consider hypoxic drive in COPD and degree of respiratory effort. Non-COPD patients should be able to maintain oxygen saturation (SpO_2) of 97% or higher. Increase oxygen concentration if SpO_2 is low.
2. Nitroglycerin SL (sublingual) is contraindicated if systolic blood pressure < 100 mm Hg and/or when the patient has taken erectile dysfunction medications within the last 72 hours.
3. History: Signs/symptoms; pain presentation, including location of pain, duration, onset, quality, relation to physical effort; history of coronary artery disease; and use of erectile dysfunction medications.
4. Right-sided myocardial infarction (MI): If you have ST elevation within V3R and/or V4R, avoid high-dose nitroglycerin. If the patient's lungs are clear, give NS 250–500 mL IV to ensure adequate ventricular-filling pressure.
5. If the ECG shows 1-mm ST elevation in two anatomically consecutive leads, contact medical command ASAP. The receiving facility may give you additional orders and will need to prepare for this patient.

Documentation

- Signs and symptoms
- Cardiac rhythm, if obtained
- Nature, intensity, and duration of pain
- Previous medical/cardiac history
- Vital signs
- SpO_2

Treatment

Response to treatment

CPR Guidelines

Response and Breathing

- If unresponsive and breathing: Place in recovery position and monitor for changes until help arrives.
- If unresponsive and not breathing (or only gasping): Check pulse for 5 to 10 seconds.
- If pulse is present open the airway and give one breath every 5 to 6 seconds. Recheck pulse every 2 minutes.
- If pulse is absent, begin chest compressions.
  - Give 30 compressions at a rate of at least 100/minute and at a depth of at least 2 inches. Allow full check recoil. Minimize interruptions in chest compressions.
- Open the airway and give two breaths that make the chest rise.
- Continue cycles of 30 compressions and 2 breaths until the AED arrives, ALS arrives, or the patient starts to move.

AED or Defibrillator Arrives

- Apply pads and analyze cardiac rhythm.
- If shock advised, deliver one shock and immediately resume CPR for 2 minutes.
- If no shock advised, immediately resume CPR for 2 minutes.
- Reanalyze cardiac rhythm every 2 minutes, deliver one shock (if indicated), and immediately resume CPR. Continue as needed until ALS arrives or the pediatric patient starts to move.

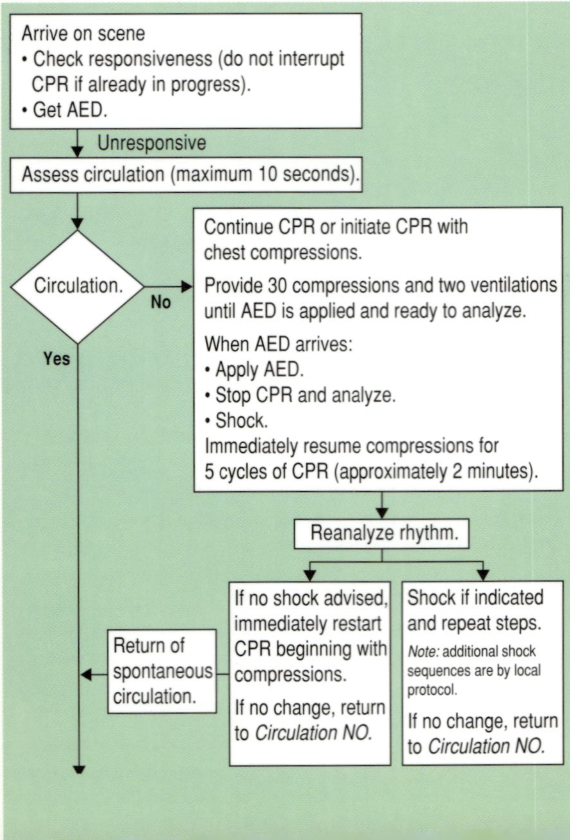
Arrive on scene
• Check responsiveness (do not interrupt CPR if already in progress).
• Get AED.
Unresponsive
Assess circulation (maximum 10 seconds).
Circulation.
No
Yes
Continue CPR or initiate CPR with chest compressions.
Provide 30 compressions and two ventilations until AED is applied and ready to analyze.
When AED arrives:
• Apply AED.
• Stop CPR and analyze.
• Shock.
Immediately resume compressions for 5 cycles of CPR (approximately 2 minutes).
Reanalyze rhythm.
If no shock advised, immediately restart CPR beginning with compressions.
If no change, return to Circulation NO.
Shock if indicated and repeat steps.
Note: additional shock sequences are by local protocol.
If no change, return to Circulation NO.
Return of spontaneous circulation.

Assess airway and breathing.
- If no clear airway, follow procedure for foreign body airway obstruction.

Breathing.

No →
- Ventilate patient every 5 to 6 seconds with supplementary oxygen and monitor the pulse.

If no pulse, return to *Circulation NO.*

Yes →
- If adequate, administer supplementary oxygen and monitor vital signs.
- If inadequate, assist ventilations, suction as needed, and monitor SpO_2 and vital signs.

Documentation

- Signs and symptoms
- Cardiac rhythm, if obtained
- Vital signs
- Oxygen saturation (SpO_2)
- Treatment
- Response to treatment

Pediatric Cardiac Arrest

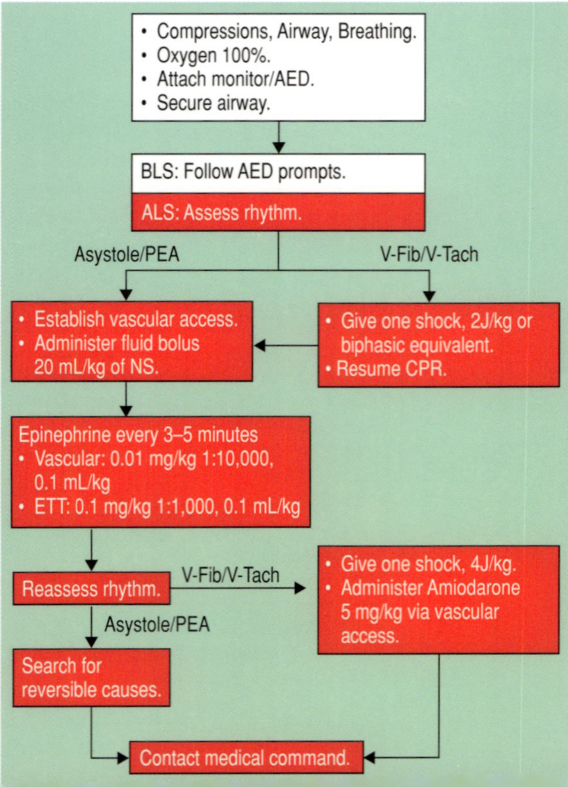

CPR

- **When intubation complete:** Rescuers no longer deliver "cycles" of CPR. Give continuous chest compressions without pauses for breaths. Give 8–10 breaths/min. Check rhythm every 2 minutes.
- **Compressions**: 100/min, ensure full chest recoil, minimize interruptions.
- **One cycle**: 15 compressions then 2 breaths.
- **Do not interrupt CPR when giving medications**.

Search for and treat reversible causes:

- Hydrogen ion (acidosis)
- Hyper/Hypokalemia
- Hypothermia
- Hypovolemia
- Hypoxia
- Tamponade, cardiac
- Tension pneumothorax
- Toxins
- Thrombosis (coronary)
- Thrombosis (pulmonary)

Pediatric Bradycardia

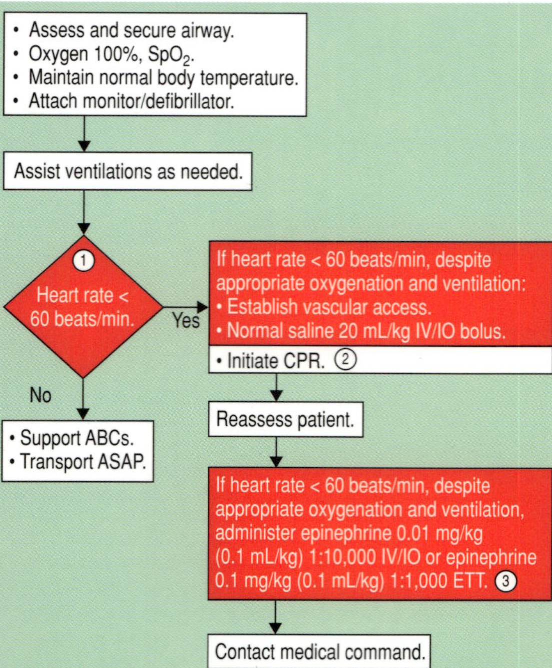

1. Heart rate < 60 beats/min with signs of cardiopulmonary compromise.

2. During CPR: Identify and treat causes: hypotension, hypovolemia, hypothermia, electrolytes, tamponade, tension pneumothorax, toxins (overdose), thromboembolism.
3. You may calculate the dose of epinephrine using a length-based resuscitation tape.

Pediatric Tachycardia

- Assess and secure airway.
- Oxygen 100%, SpO_2.
- Maintain normal body temperature.
- Attach monitor/defibrillator.

↓

- Establish vascular access.
- Normal saline 20 mL/kg IV/IO bolus.

↓

Narrow complex. (1)

↓

If rhythm is regular and patient is hemodynamically stable, attempt vagal maneuvers.

↓

Wide complex.

↓

Contact medical command.

continues

↓

If conscious and rhythm is regular (probably not sinus tachycardia), administer adenosine 0.1 mg/kg rapid IV/IO push followed by 10 mL normal saline bolus.

↓

If no conversion, and rhythm is not A-fib or A-flutter, and no history of Wolf Parkinson White, administer:
adenosine 0.2 mg/kg rapid IV/IO push followed by 10 mL normal saline bolus.

↓

Contact medical command.

1. Narrow complex tachycardia that is likely supraventricular in etiology.

Advanced Cardiac Life Support

The following protocols are for adults only.

Asystole and PEA

- Start or continue CPR: 5 cycles (30 chest compressions and 2 ventilations per cycle).
- Oxygen, SpO_2.
- Attach cardiac monitor/defibrillator. If asystole, confirm in a second lead.

↓

Secure an airway.

↓

- Establish vascular access without interrupting CPR.
- Administer fluid bolus.
- Epinephrine 1 mg 1:10,000 IV/IO or 2 mg 1:10,000 ETT every 3–5 minutes double dose same strength, or administer vasopressin 40 units IV/IO. (1) (2)

↓

Search for and treat reversible causes:

- Hydrogen ion (acidosis)
- Hyper/Hypokalemia
- Hypothermia
- Hypovolemia
- Hypoxia
- Tamponade, cardiac
- Tension pneumothorax
- Toxins
- Thrombosis (coronary)
- Thrombosis (pulmonary)

↓

continues

- Contact medical command.
- Consider termination of efforts ONLY with the input of the medical command physician if asystole/agonal rhythms continue after advanced airway placement and initial medications and no reversible causes are identified. The time interval since onset of arrest shall be considered.

CPR

- When intubation complete: Rescuers no longer deliver "cycles" of CPR. Give continuous chest compressions without pauses for breaths. Give 8–10 breaths/min.
- Compressions: at least 100/min, push hard (2 inches), allow full chest recoil, minimize interruptions.
- Prior to advanced airway: 30 compressions, then 2 breaths.
- Do not interrupt CPR when giving medications.

1. The choice between epinephrine and vasopressin shall be at the discretion of the program's medical director. Vasopressin may be used in place of epinephrine first or second dose.
2. ETT: The total amount of solutions given via ETT is not to exceed 50 mL.

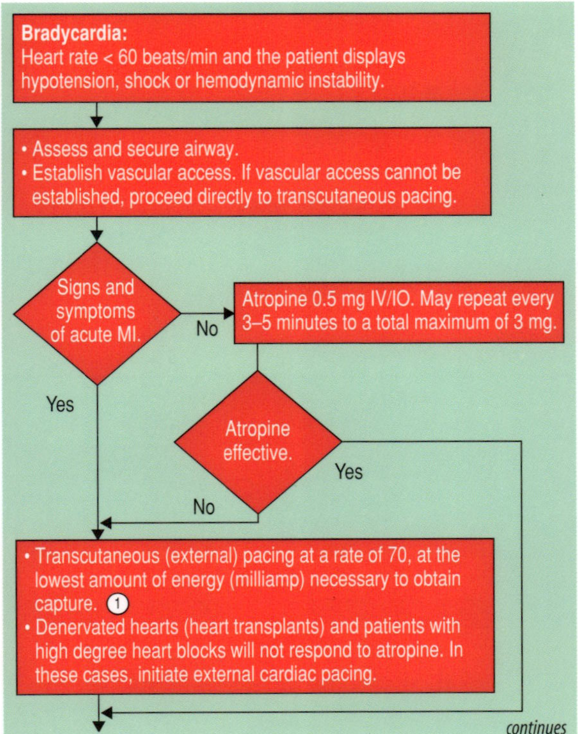
Bradycardia:
Heart rate < 60 beats/min and the patient displays hypotension, shock or hemodynamic instability.
• Assess and secure airway.
• Establish vascular access. If vascular access cannot be established, proceed directly to transcutaneous pacing.
Signs and symptoms of acute MI.
No
Atropine 0.5 mg IV/IO. May repeat every 3–5 minutes to a total maximum of 3 mg.
Yes
Atropine effective.
Yes
No
• Transcutaneous (external) pacing at a rate of 70, at the lowest amount of energy (milliamp) necessary to obtain capture. (1)
• Denervated hearts (heart transplants) and patients with high degree heart blocks will not respond to atropine. In these cases, initiate external cardiac pacing.

continues

- Contact medical command.
- In stable patients with Type II second degree or third degree AV block, external pacemaker should be applied as a precaution.

Search for and treat reversible causes:

- Hydrogen ion (acidosis)
- Hyper/Hypokalemia
- Hypothermia
- Hypovolemia
- Hypoxia
- Tamponade, cardiac
- Tension pneumothorax
- Toxins
- Thrombosis (coronary)
- Thrombosis (pulmonary)

1. Consider sedation with Lorazepam 0.05 mg/kg to a maximum of 2 mg or Midazolam 0.05 mg/kg to a maximum of 5 mg.

Ventricular Fibrillation and Pulseless Ventricular Tachycardia

- If NOT a witnessed arrest, start or continue CPR for 5 cycles (30 compressions and 2 ventilations per cycle).
- If CPR has been started by a first responder or witnessed arrest by ALS crew member, immediately review the cardiac rhythm. If indicated, defibrillate at 360 J or biphasic equivalent and immediately resume CPR.

↓

During CPR:

- Assess and secure airway.
- Establish vascular access and administer fluid bolus.
- Epinephrine 1 mg 1:10,000 IV/IO or 2 mg 1:10,000 ETT every 3–5 minutes up to a total of 3 doses, or administer vasopressin 40 units IV/IO one time only and continue CPR. (1)

↓

Reassess rhythm every 2 minutes. If rhythm remains V-Fib or pulseless V-Tach:

- Defibrillate 360 J or equivalent biphasic and immediately resume CPR for 5 cycles.
- If at any time the patient has a return of spontaneous circulation and has NOT been given an anti-dysrhythmic medication, administer amiodarone 150 mg IV/IO over 10 minutes.

↓

continues

↓

During CPR:
- Amiodarone 300 mg IV/IO and continue CPR.

↓

Contact medical command.

↓

If V-Fib/Pulseless V-Tach recur after contact with medical command, an ALS crew member may repeat entire protocol until medical command can be recontacted.

CPR
- **When intubation complete:** Rescuers no longer deliver "cycles" of CPR. Give continuous chest compressions without pauses for breaths. Give 8–10 breaths/min.
- **Compressions:** at least 100/min, push hard ($\geq$ 2 inches), allow full recoil, minimize interruptions.
- **Prior to advanced airway:** 30 compressions, then 2 breaths.
- **Do not interrupt CPR when giving medications**.

Search for and treat reversible causes:

- Hydrogen ion (acidosis)
- Hyper/Hypokalemia
- Hypothermia
- Hypovolemia
- Hypoxia
- Tamponade, cardiac
- Tension pneumothorax
- Toxins
- Thrombosis (coronary)
- Thrombosis (pulmonary)

1. ETT: The total amount of solutions given via ETT is not to exceed 50 mL.

Tachycardia

Narrow Complex Tachycardia—Stable

- Airway.
- Oxygen, SpO_2.
- Establish vascular access.
- Monitor and identify cardiac rhythm and vital signs.

↓

- Patient assessment, medical history, allergies.
- Perform a 12-lead ECG.

↓

Wolf Parkinson White present.

Yes → Contact medical command.

No ↓

- Attempt vagal maneuvers.
- Adenosine 6 mg rapid IV over 1–3 seconds followed immediately by a rapid 20 mL IV bolus of normal saline.

↓

A-Fib or A-Flutter identified.

Yes → Diltiazem (Cardiazem) 0.25 mg/kg IV over 2 minutes.

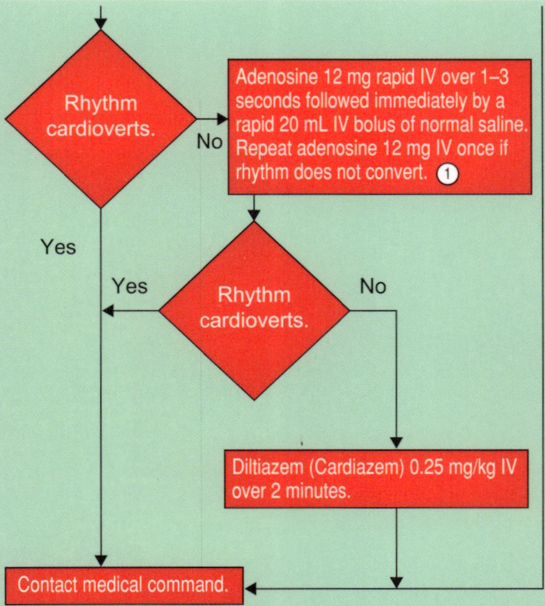

1. If A-Fib or A-Flutter is identified at any time and no Wolf Parkinson White is known or suspected, administer diltiazem (Cardiazem) 0.25 mg/kg IV over two minutes and contact medical command. (Do not give two doses of Cardiazem.)

Narrow Complex Tachycardia—Unstable

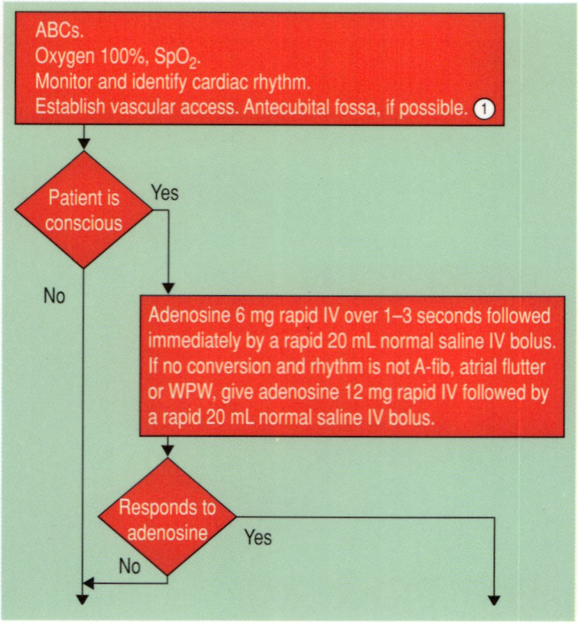

Synchronized cardioversion at 50 J or equivalent biphasic. Check pulse/rhythm after shock. (2)

If the rhythm fails to convert, perform a synchronized cardioversion at **100 J** or equivalent biphasic. Check pulse/rhythm after shock.

If the rhythm fails to convert, perform a synchronized cardioversion at **200 J** or equivalent biphasic. Check pulse/rhythm after shock.

If the rhythm fails to convert, perform a synchronized cardioversion at **300 J** or equivalent biphasic. Check pulse/rhythm after shock.

If the rhythm fails to convert, perform a synchronized cardioversion at **360 J** or equivalent biphasic. Check pulse/rhythm after shock.

Contact medical command.

continues

1. If unable to establish vascular access, perform a synchronized cardioversion as outlined in protocol.
2. If the patient is conscious, administer sedation if appropriate. Lorazepam (Ativan) 0.05 mg/kg up to 2 mg or midazolam (Versed) 0.05 mg/kg up to 5 mg.

Ventricular Tachycardia with Pulses—Stable ①

- ABCs.
- Oxygen, SpO_2.
- 12-lead ECG.
- Monitor vital signs.
- Establish vascular access.

↓

If sustained wide-complex tachycardia, administer amiodarone 150 mg IV over 10 minutes.

↓

Contact medical command.

1. Stable ventricular tachycardia: The patient's systolic blood pressure is greater than or equal to 90 mm Hg.

Ventricular Tachycardia with Pulses—Unstable ①

- ABCs.
- Oxygen 100%, SpO_2.
- Monitor and identify cardiac rhythm. ②
- Establish vascular access.

Patient is conscious

Yes → If the patient is conscious, administer sedation if appropriate. Lorazepam (Ativan) 0.05 mg/kg up to 2 mg or midazolam (Versed) 0.05 mg/kg up to 5 mg.

No ↓

Synchronized cardioversion at 100 J or equivalent biphasic. Check pulse/rhythm after shock. ③

↓

If the rhythm fails to convert, synchronized cardioversion at **200 J** or equivalent biphasic. Check pulse/rhythm after shock.

↓

If the rhythm fails to convert, synchronized cardioversion at **300 J** or equivalent biphasic. Check pulse/rhythm after shock

↓

If the rhythm fails to convert, synchronized cardioversion at **360 J** or equivalent biphasic. Check pulse/rhythm after shock.

↓

Contact medical command.

1. Unstable wide-complex tachycardia where the patient is unconscious or hemodynamically compromised.
2. If a patient presents with polymorphic V-Tach and is unstable, treat the rhythm as V-Fib and deliver high-energy, unsynchronized shocks at 360 J or biphasic equivalent. If there is any doubt whether monomorphic or polymorphic V-Tach is present in the unstable patient, do not delay shock delivery to perform detailed rhythm analysis—provide high-energy unsynchronized shocks (i.e. defibrillation doses).
3. If the rhythm converts at any point, administer amiodarone 150 mg IV/IO over 10 minutes.

Documentation

- Detailed assessment
- Cardiac rhythm
- Chief complaint
- Treatment
- Response to treatment
- Vital signs
- Oxygen saturation (SpO_2)
- Lung sounds
- Level of consciousness
- Verification of ET tube placement or use of airway adjuncts
- Communication with medical command physician

Normal Delivery Childbirth

Considerations

Transport to a facility with obstetric capabilities for abnormal presentation.

Gravid: The total number of pregnancies, not necessarily carried to term.

Para: The total number of pregnancies carried to more than 28 weeks' gestation, regardless of whether delivered dead or alive.

Assessment

- Airway, breathing, circulation.
- Administer 100% oxygen.
- BLS to request ALS.
- If the baby is NOT crowning, transport the patient on her left side and rendezvous with ALS.
- If the baby is crowning, do not transport. Prepare for delivery.
- If foot, hand, cord, or face presents, place in Trendelenburg position, prevent cord compression with gloved hand, and transport ASAP.
- **If normal presentation exists**, control the delivery of the head. Support head during rotation. Bulb suction mouth, then nose. Guide head down to deliver the anterior shoulder, then upward to deliver the posterior shoulder. Control delivery of trunk and legs. The trunk and legs are often released quickly after the shoulders are delivered. Anticipate this and control their delivery. Clamp cord 8 inches from the navel twice, 2 inches apart. Cut between the clamps.
- Treat the baby per neonatal resuscitation program guidelines. Keep the baby warm.
- Perform APGAR scores at 1, 5, and 10 minutes.
- Record time of birth.
- Transport mother and baby.

- Watch for delivery of placenta. Do not pull on the cord. Document time the placenta delivers.
- If significant vaginal bleeding is present, intermittently massage the fundus until it is firm. Expedite transport.

Treatment

- ABCs.
- Oxygen, SpO_2.
- ALS: Establish vascular access.

↓

History and exam: ① ②
Previous births, prenatal care, edema, multiple births, previous C-section, medical history, vital signs, frequency of contractions, fetal heart rate.

↓

Crowning.

Yes → Prepare for delivery. ↓

No → Position lateral recumbent. ↓

- Transport to most appropriate facility.
- Monitor vital signs.
- Comfort.

continues

Treatment, continued

Control delivery of head.
Support head with rotation.

↓

Suction mouth, then nose with bulb suction.

↓

Guide head down to deliver anterior shoulder, then upward to deliver posterior shoulder.

↓

Control delivery of trunk and legs.

↓

Clamp cord 8 inches from navel, 2 inches apart, and cut between clamps.

↓

- Treat baby per neonatal resuscitation program guidelines.
- Perform APGAR score at 1, 5, 10 minutes.
- Keep baby warm.
- Note time of birth.

↓

Watch for delivery of placenta. Do not pull on cord. After delivery of placenta, intermittently massage fundus until firm.

↓

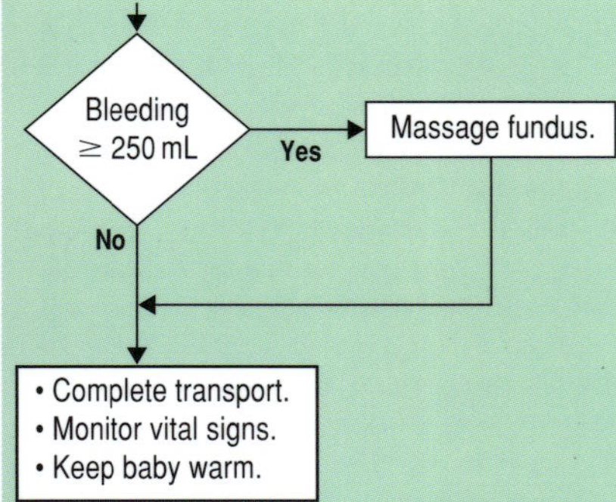

1. Normal fetal heart rate is 120 to 150 beats/min.
2. Do NOT perform a digital cervical examination. Because of the possibilities of placental previa or abruptio placenta, digital cervical exams are contraindicated.

Documentation

- Maternal history: gravida ____; para ____
- Gestational age in weeks/days
- Estimated date of conception
- Frequency and duration of contractions
- Time of birth
- APGAR score at 1, 5, and 10 minutes
- Time of placental delivery
- Estimated fluid/blood loss
- Complications, if any
- Communication with medical command, if any

Abnormal Delivery Childbirth

Considerations

Transport to a facility with obstetric capabilities for abnormal presentation.

Gravid: The total number of pregnancies, not necessarily carried to term.

Para: The total number of pregnancies carried to more than 28 weeks' gestation, regardless of whether delivered dead or alive.

Assessment

- Airway, breathing, circulation.
- Administer 100% oxygen.
- BLS to request ALS.
- If the baby is NOT crowning, transport the patient on her left side and rendezvous with ALS.
- If the baby is crowning, do not transport. Prepare for delivery.
- If foot, hand, cord, or face presents, place in Trendelenburg position, prevent cord compression with gloved hand, and transport ASAP.
- If breech presentation (buttocks), support legs and trunk as they deliver. Do not pull on the baby. Deliver arms before the head. Lower body to help head deliver. As hairline appears, move chin to chest. Head should deliver. If there is a delay in delivery while in a breech presentation and the baby attempts to breathe, form a V with your fingers and hold the vaginal wall away from the baby's face, allowing the baby to breathe. Suction mouth, then nose.
- If the umbilical cord is wrapped around the baby's neck, slip the cord over the head. If this is not possible, place two clamps 2 inches apart, cut the cord, and remove the cord from the baby's neck.
- Treat the baby per neonatal resuscitation program guidelines. Keep the baby warm.
- Perform APGAR scores at 1, 5, and 10 minutes.
- Record time of birth.

- Transport mother and baby.
- Watch for delivery of placenta. Do not pull on the cord. Document time the placenta delivers.
- If significant vaginal bleeding is present, intermittently massage the fundus until it is firm. Expedite transport.

Treatment

- ABCs.
- Oxygen, SpO_2.
- Establish vascular access.

↓

Breech presentation. ①

↓

Foot, hand, cord, face present.

Yes →

- Place patient in Trendelenburg position.
- Prevent cord compression with gloved hand.

↓

- Transport ASAP.
- Monitor vital signs.

No ↓

Buttocks presentation. ②

↓

Position the mother with her buttocks at the edge of the bed with her legs flexed.

↓

continues

Treatment, continued

↓

Allow the baby's buttocks and trunk to deliver spontaneously. Do not pull on the baby.

↓

When the baby's legs clear, support the body on the palm of your hand and the anterior forearm.

↓

Lower the baby slightly. This will help the head pass through the pelvic outlet.

↓

When the baby's hairline appears, grasp the baby's ankles and lift him upward toward the mother's abdomen. The head should deliver easily.

Prolapsed umbilical cord.

↓

Position the mother with her hips elevated as much as possible. Administer oxygen 100%. Instruct the woman to pant with each contraction to prevent pushing. With your gloved hand, gently push the baby (not the cord) back up into the vagina until the presenting part no longer presses against the cord. You must maintain this position throughout urgent transport to the hospital.

Cord around the neck.

↓

Slip cord over head or place clamps 2 inches apart and cut cord, then unwrap from neck.

↓

Bulb suction mouth, then nose.

1. **Breech presentation:** When a body part other than the baby's head presents first.
2. **Buttocks presentation:** If the baby's head does not deliver within 3 minutes, the baby is in danger of suffocating. Immediately place your gloved hand in the vagina, with your palm toward the baby's face. Form a V with your fingers on either side of the baby's nose and push the vaginal wall away from the baby's face until the head is delivered. If the baby's head does not deliver within 3 minutes of providing an airway, provide rapid transport to the hospital, with the mother's buttocks elevated on pillows. Maintain the baby's airway throughout transport. Alert the hospital so they can have the appropriate personnel on hand when the mother arrives.

Documentation

- Maternal history: gravida _____, para ______
- Gestational age in weeks/days
- Estimated date of conception
- Frequency and duration of contractions
- Time of birth
- APGAR score at 1, 5, and 10 minutes
- Time of placental delivery
- Estimated fluid/blood loss
- Complications
- Communication with medical command

Pregnancy Bleeding

Considerations

Abruptio placenta: The premature separation of a normally implanted placenta from the wall of the uterus. The patient usually reports vaginal bleeding, with bright red blood. The patient almost always reports sudden and severe abdominal pain. The abdomen is tender and rigid. Shock is often significant.

Placenta previa: The placenta is implanted low in the uterus, and as it grows it partially or completely obscures the cervical canal. This is the leading cause of vaginal bleeding in the second and third trimester. Typical signs and symptoms include painless vaginal bleeding with a loss of bright red blood. The uterus is soft and nontender. Do not try to palpate the abdomen deeply.

Eclampsia: A disorder that may occur in late pregnancy, during or immediately after childbirth, that is characterized by seizures, edema, hypertension, and proteinuria. Suspect/assume preeclampsia or eclampsia if the pregnant patient has an elevated blood pressure.

Assessment

- Airway, breathing, circulation.
- Administer 100% oxygen.
- BLS to request ALS.
- Transport ASAP.
- Place in lateral recumbent position, if in second or third trimester.
- Do not attempt to perform a digital, internal vaginal exam or pack the vagina with trauma pads.
- Do not try to palpate the abdomen deeply. Deep or firm palpation may induce heavy vaginal bleeding.

Treatment

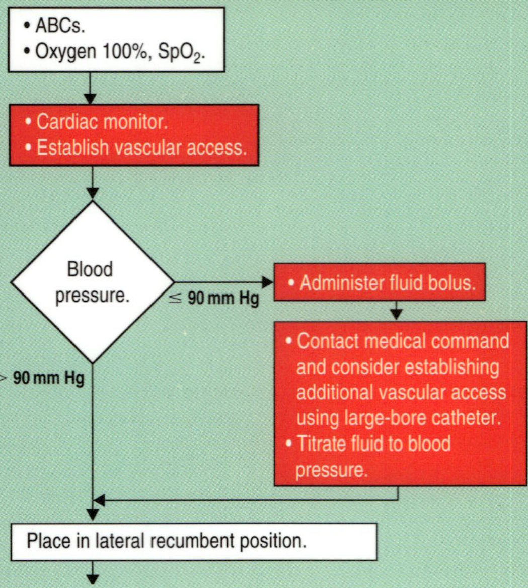
• ABCs.
• Oxygen 100%, SpO_2.
• Cardiac monitor.
• Establish vascular access.
Blood pressure.
≤ 90 mm Hg
• Administer fluid bolus.
• Contact medical command and consider establishing additional vascular access using large-bore catheter.
• Titrate fluid to blood pressure.
> 90 mm Hg
Place in lateral recumbent position.

↓

Do **NOT** perform internal digital exam or attempt to palpate abdomen deeply/firmly.

↓

- Keep patient warm.
- Provide supportive care.
- Preserve tissue fragments.
- Notify receiving hospital ASAP.

Documentation

- Signs and symptoms
- Oxygen saturation (SpO_2)
- Cardiac rhythm
- Time bleeding started
- Estimated amount of bleeding
- Nature of pain, if present (dull, sharp, cramping, duration, frequency)
- Color of blood

Neonatal Resuscitation

Assessment

- BLS to request ALS.
- Keep baby warm.
- Position, clear airway.
- Suction mouth, then nose.
- Provide gentle tactile stimulation.
- Dry, then stimulate to breathe.
- Assess respirations, heart rate, and skin color:
  - If apneic or heart rate is < 100 beats/min, provide positive-pressure ventilation. If heart rate is > 60 beats/min, begin chest compressions.
  - If breathing and heart rate is >100 beats/min and skin is cyanotic, give 100% oxygen blow-by. If cyanosis persists, provide positive-pressure ventilation. If the infant becomes pink, is breathing, and heart rate is >100 beats/min, observe closely and transport ASAP.
  - If breathing and heart rate is >100 beats/min and skin is pink, observe closely and transport ASAP.

Term Newborn Vital Signs

Heart rate (awake): 100-180 beats/min
Respiratory rate: 30-60 breaths/min
Systolic blood pressure: 55-90 mm Hg
Diastolic blood pressure: 26-55 mm Hg

Treatment

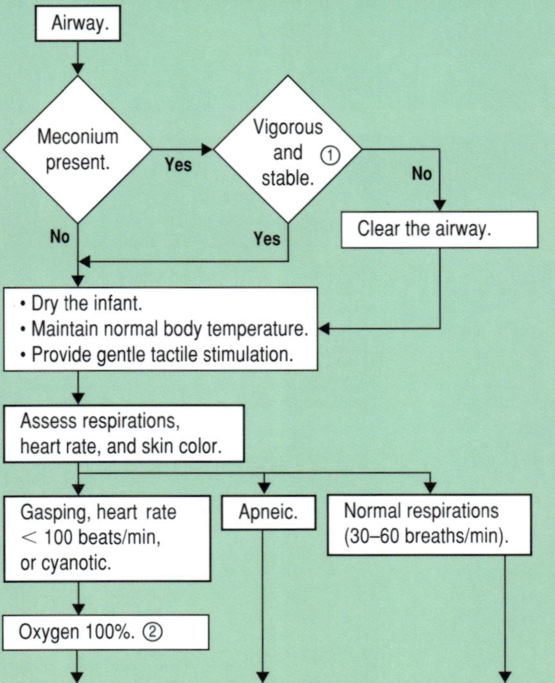

continues

Treatment, continued

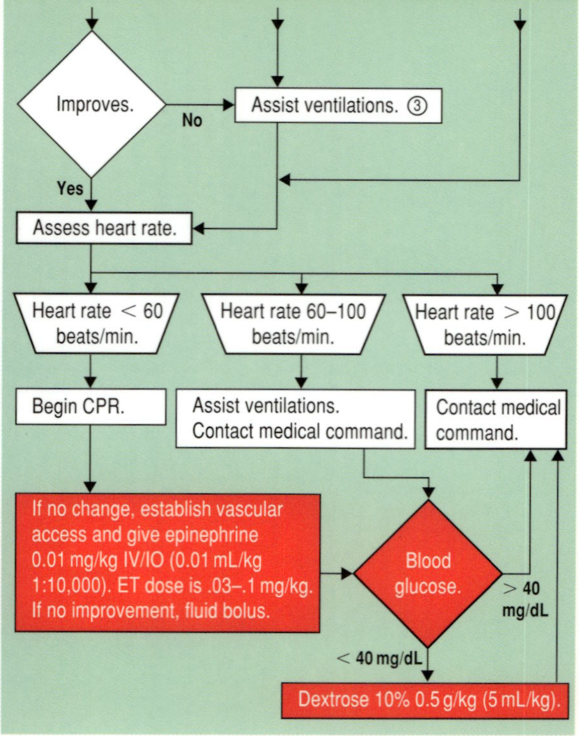

1. Vigorous and stable: strong respiratory effort, good muscle tone, and heart rate of 100 beats/min or greater.
2. Give lower concentrations of oxygen if the neonate is premature. In general, neonates should not be on long-term high concentrations of oxygen.
3. Begin bag-valve-mask ventilations at a rate of 40-60 breaths/min with sufficient volume to cause visible chest expansion. Reassess every 30 seconds.

Pediatric Considerations

ALS: Medications Used in Neonatal Resuscitation

- Epinephrine 1:10,000: 0.01 mg/kg IV/IO.
- Normal Saline: Fluid bolus of 20 mL/kg over 5-10 minutes. Indicated for shock.
- Sodium Bicarbonate: 1-2 mEq/kg IV over 2 minutes. Use only in prolonged resuscitation and when infant is effectively ventilated.
- Naloxone (Narcan): 0.1 mg/kg IV or IM. Establish adequate ventilation first. Give rapidly. Use cautiously in opioid-addicted mothers.
- Dextrose 10%: 0.5 g/kg (5 mL/kg) slow IV. Check bedside blood glucose.

Documentation

- Respiratory effort and quality
- Skin color
- Capillary refill
- Response to treatment
- APGAR scores at 1, 5 and 10 minutes

CNS Depressant

Considerations

Potential signs and symptoms of depressant use include central nervous system (CNS) and respiratory depression, drowsiness, nausea, vomiting, pinpoint pupils, and bradycardia.

Assessment

- Airway, breathing, circulation.
- Administer 100% oxygen.
- Assist ventilations, as needed.
- BLS to request ALS.
- Transport ASAP.

Treatment

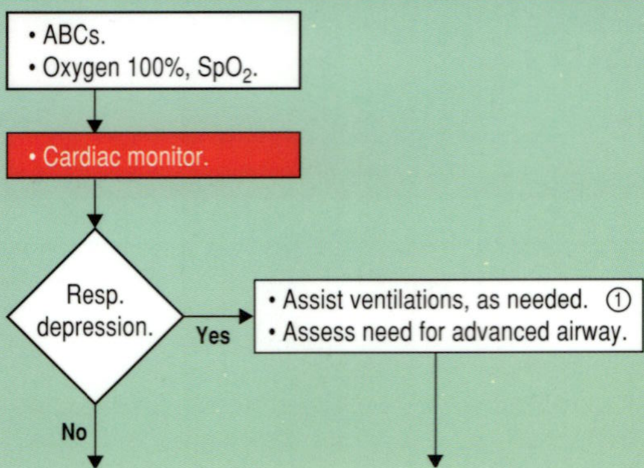

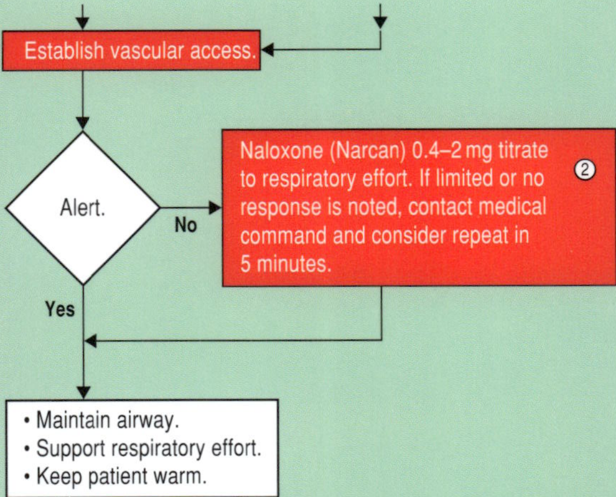

1. Consider administering naloxone (Narcan) (while assisting ventilations) before inserting an advanced airway. A brief trial of naloxone (Narcan) may quickly reverse the patient's condition and eliminate the need for an advanced airway.
2. Naloxone (Narcan): Duration 30–60 minutes. Be prepared to repeat treatment, because the effect of naloxone (Narcan) may wear off. Anticipate a rapid onset. Be prepared to restrain combative and/or confused patients. Titrate to respiratory effort. Use with caution in narcotic-dependent patients and neonates of narcotic-dependent mothers.

Pediatric Considerations

ALS

Naloxone (Narcan) dose: 0.1 mg/kg/dose IV, IM. Maximum dose: 2 mg. If no response in 10 minutes, administer a second dose 0.1 mg/kg.

Documentation

- Signs and symptoms
- Glasgow Coma Scale (GCS) score
- Response to treatment
- Oxygen saturation (SpO_2)
- Cardiac rhythm, if obtained

Tricyclic Antidepressant

Considerations

- Potential signs and symptoms of tricyclic antidepressant overdose include: wide QRS, tachycardia, ventricular dysrhythmias, hypoventilation, decreased level of consciousness (LOC), seizures, cardiovascular collapse, dry, flushed (red) skin, and hypotension.
- Tricyclics include: amitriptyline (Amitril, Elavil, Endep, Emitrip, Enovil, Etrafon, Limbitrol, Triavil); amoxapine (Asendin, Asendis, Defanyl, Demolox, Moxadil); desipramine (Norpamin, Pertofane); doxepin (Aponal, Sinaquan); imipramine (Antideprin, Deprimin, Tofranil); maprotiline (Deprilept, Ludiomil); nortriptyline (Aventyl, Pamelor); protriptyline (Vivactil); trimipramine (Surmontil).

Assessment

- Airway, breathing, circulation.
- Administer 100% oxygen.
- Assist ventilations, as needed.
- BLS to request ALS if ANY of the signs and/or symptoms are present.
- RAPID transport ASAP.

Treatment

- ABCs.
- Oxygen, SpO_2.
- Assist ventilations, as needed.
- Advanced airway, as needed.

↓

- Cardiac monitor.
- Establish vascular access.

↓

continues

Treatment, continued

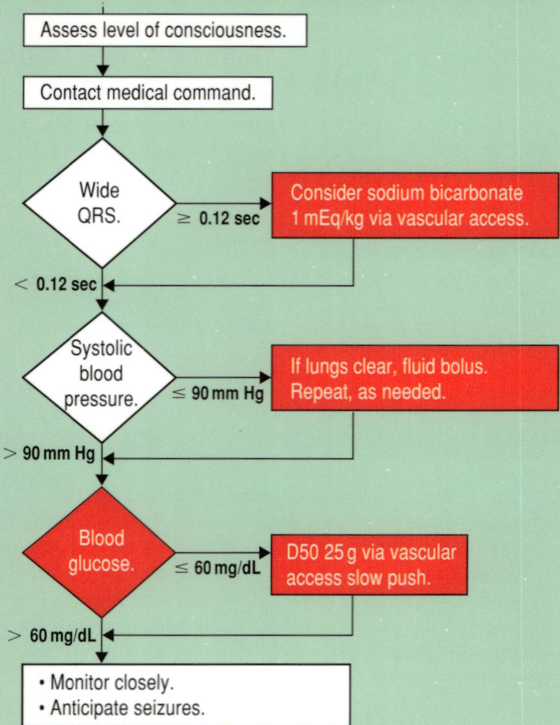

Pediatric Considerations

ALS

Dextrose: Patients younger than 1 month, administer dextrose 10% (D10) solution 0.5 g/kg slow IV/IO; patients 1 month or older, administer dextrose 25% (D25) solution, 0.5 g/kg slow IV/IO.

Documentation

- Signs and symptoms
- Glasgow Coma Scale (GCS) score
- Response to treatment
- Oxygen saturation (SpO_2)
- Cardiac rhythm

Asthma

Considerations

The absence of normal lung sounds strongly suggests the patient is moving little to no air. Respiratory arrest may be imminent.

Assessment

- Airway, breathing, circulation.
- Administer 100% oxygen.
- Transport ASAP.
- BLS to consider ALS backup.
- Allow patient to sit in a position of comfort.
- Maintain body temperature.
- **BLS: Metered dose inhaler (MDI) administration:** You may assist the patient to administer a rescue inhaler if:
  - The patient possesses his or her own prescribed MDI,
  - AND the patient is alert enough to use the inhaler properly,
  - AND the patient has NOT taken the maximum number of inhalations per the prescription.

Procedure for MDI Administration

1. Check the medication's expiration date. Do not assist with the inhaler if it is beyond the expiration date.
2. Remove the oxygen delivery device from the patient's face.
3. Instruct the patient to exhale deeply.
4. Have the patient assist by placing his or her lips around the mouthpiece of the inhaler. Note: If the patient has a spacer device for use with the inhaler, it should be used.
5. Assist the patient in depressing the cartridge as he or she takes a deep inhalation.
6. Instruct the patient to hold his or her breath for as long as possible.
7. Replace the oxygen delivery device to the patient's face.

8. Allow the patient to breathe a few times before assessing the need to administer an additional dose.
9. Do not delay transport.

Treatment

- ABCs.
- Oxygen 100%, SpO_2 ①
- Assist ventilations, as needed.

↓

Respiratory distress.

Yes →

- Assist patient with prescribed rescue inhaler. See *Assessment* section for guidelines.
- ALS: Albuterol (Proventil) 2.5 mg and ipratropium bromide 0.5 mg in NS via nebulizer. ②

↓

- Monitor cardiac rhythm.
- Establish vascular access.

↓

For pediatric patients: If patient becomes unstable consider epinephrine 0.01 mg/kg of 1:1,000 to max of 0.05 mg IM.

↓

No ↓

continues

Contact medical command.

Reassess vital signs, SpO_2, respiratory status.

1. If chronic obstructive pulmonary disease (COPD) coexists, titrate oxygen to maintain $SpO_2 > 90\%$.
2. Albuterol (Proventil): May administer up to two additional albuterol (Proventil) 2.5 mg via nebulizer.

Pediatric Considerations

ALS

- Administer albuterol (Proventil) 2.5 mg and ipratropium bromide 0.5 mg in 3 mL normal saline via nebulizer.
- Administer additional albuterol 2.5 mg in 3 mL normal saline via nebulizer, up to a total of three treatments.
- Contact medical command.

Documentation

- Respiratory effort
- Lung sounds before/after airway management
- Oxygen saturation (SpO_2), capnography
- Treatment
- Response to treatment
- Skin color
- Glasgow Coma Scale (GCS) score

Chronic Obstructive Pulmonary Disease (COPD)

Considerations

- The absence of lung sounds strongly suggests the patient is moving little to no air. Respiratory arrest may be imminent.
- **Hypoxic drive:** A healthy patient exhales because the body detects the presence of carbon dioxide. Some patients with chronic obstructive pulmonary disease (COPD), unlike healthy patients, use their hypoxic drive (exhale/inhale because their body detects lower oxygen level). When COPD patients who are using their hypoxic drive are given too much oxygen, their respiratory drive may decrease or stop when their body detects ample oxygen. As a result, expect and accept oxygen saturation (SpO_2) readings below 90% and above 85% on patients with COPD. Give lower concentrations (2–3 L/min via nasal cannula) to these patients, but never deprive a patient in respiratory distress of oxygen. If a patient is in respiratory distress, give high concentrations of oxygen.

Assessment

- Airway, breathing, circulation.
- Administer oxygen 2 L/min via nasal cannula. If symptoms do not improve, switch to a nonrebreathing mask. Assist ventilations, as needed.
- Assist the patient with use of any prescribed metered-dose inhalers (MDI) he or she may have.
- Transport ASAP.
- BLS to consider ALS.
- Allow patient to sit up in a position of comfort.
- BLS: Complaints of respiratory distress and wheezing, assist patient with their own MDI, not to exceed maximum prescribed dose.

Treatment

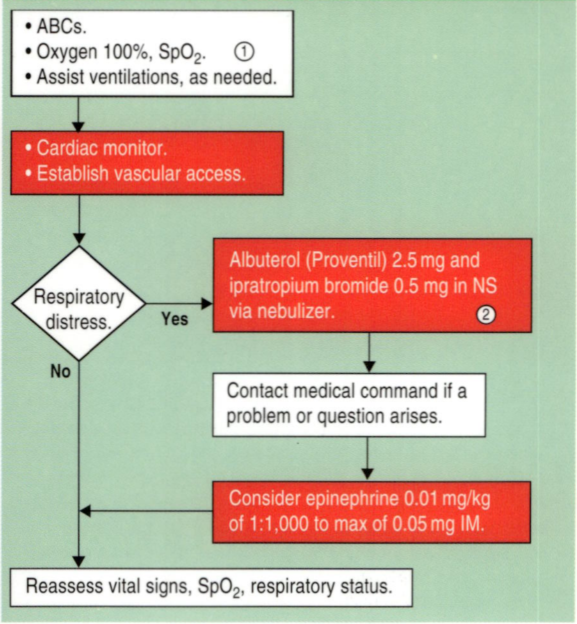
• ABCs.
• Oxygen 100%, SpO2. ①
• Assist ventilations, as needed.
• Cardiac monitor.
• Establish vascular access.
Respiratory distress.
Yes
No
Albuterol (Proventil) 2.5 mg and ipratropium bromide 0.5 mg in NS via nebulizer. ②
Contact medical command if a problem or question arises.
Consider epinephrine 0.01 mg/kg of 1:1,000 to max of 0.05 mg IM.
Reassess vital signs, SpO2, respiratory status.

1. Oxygen: Adjust flow rate and route of administration, as needed. Consider hypoxic drive in COPD and degree of respiratory effort. A target SpO_2 of 90% is ideal. Avoid higher SpO_2 readings unless patient is in severe or moderate distress. If symptoms do not improve, switch to a nonrebreathing mask. Assist ventilations, as needed.
2. Albuterol (Proventil): May administer up to three total doses. Discontinue use if patient develops chest pain or increased tachycardia. First dose of albuterol (Proventil) may be combined with ipratropium bromide (Atrovent).

Documentation

- Respiratory effort
- Lung sounds before/after airway management
- Oxygen saturation (SpO_2), capnography
- Treatment
- Response to treatment
- Skin color
- Glasgow Coma Scale (GCS) score

Congestive Heart Failure (CHF)

Considerations

- The absence of lung sounds strongly suggests the patient is moving little to no air. Respiratory arrest may be imminent.
- It is often difficult to differentiate congestive heart failure (CHF) from chronic obstructive pulmonary disease (COPD). When in doubt, ask the patient what medications he or she is taking. Patients taking digoxin and/or furosemide (Lasix) are probably being treated for CHF.
- Possible signs and symptoms: Dyspnea, rales, wheezing, frothy-pink sputum, jugular vein distention, peripheral edema.
- If in respiratory distress, consider CPAP.

Assessment

- Airway, breathing, circulation.
- Administer oxygen, as needed.
- Assist ventilations, as needed.
- Transport ASAP.
- BLS to consider ALS.
- Allow patient to sit up in a position of comfort.
- If chest pain is present, consider assisting the patient with his or her prescribed nitroglycerin.

Treatment

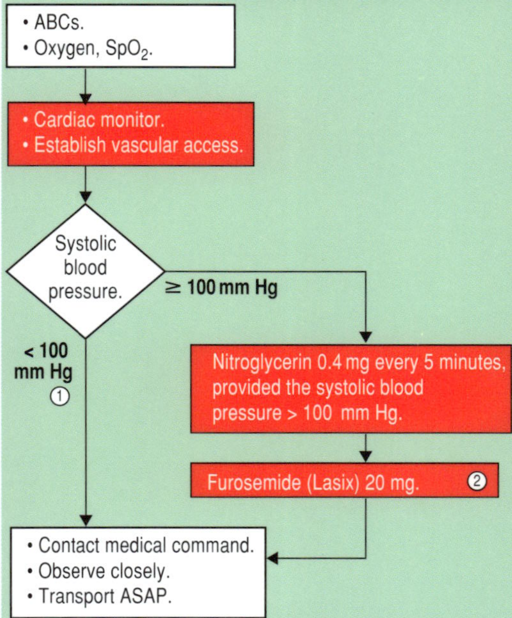

1. Consider dopamine if blood pressure is < 100 mm Hg.
2. A provider's medical director may elect to substitute bumetanide (Bumex) 0.5 mg for furosemide (Lasix).

Documentation

- Respiratory effort
- Lung sounds before/after airway management
- Oxygen saturation (SpO_2), capnography
- Treatment
- Response to treatment
- Skin color
- Glasgow Coma Scale (GCS) score

Croup and Epiglottitis

Considerations

- Approach the child in a calm and reassuring manner. Do not startle the patient; anxiety is likely to exacerbate the patient.
- Allow the child to adopt position of comfort.
- Consider blow-by humidified oxygen. Pediatric patients rarely tolerate a mask.
- Mild to moderate distress: Barking cough, inspiratory stridor.
- Moderate to severe distress: Stridor at rest, retractions, tripoding, and accessory muscle use.
- Children who have not had immunization are at a greater risk for acute epiglottitis.

Croup

- Age 6 months through 3 years.
- Gradual onset.
- Signs and symptoms: Often preceded by an upper respiratory infection.
- Often worse at night.
- May or may not have a fever.
- Condition varies from mild to severe.

Epiglottitis

- Age usually > 2 years.
- Rapid onset.
- Sign and symptoms: Fever, often looks sick, air hunger, nasal flaring, restlessness, drooling, retractions, wants to sit upright.

Assessment

- Airway, breathing, circulation.
- Administer 100% oxygen. Consider blow-by humidified oxygen (pediatric patients rarely tolerate mask).
- Assist ventilations, as needed.
- Maintain body temperature.
- Monitor cardiac rhythm.
- BLS to consider ALS.
- Transport ASAP.

Treatment

- Approach the child in a calm, reassuring fashion.
- Allow the child to adopt position of comfort.
- Transport with parent/guardian, if possible. ①

↓

- Maintain airway.
- Oxygen 100%, SpO_2. ②

↓

- Cardiac monitor.
- Establish vascular access (if medically necessary).

↓

Mild to moderate distress.

Yes → Administer NS 3 mL nebulized with simple mask and contact medical command.

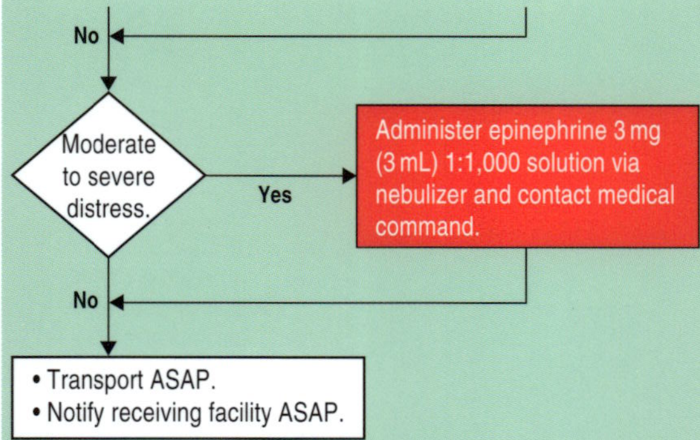

1. Avoid startling the child. Anxiety is likely to exacerbate the child's condition.
2. Consider blow-by oxygen. Pediatric patients rarely tolerate a mask.

Documentation

- Respiratory effort
- Lung sounds before/after airway management
- Oxygen saturation (SpO_2)
- Treatment
- Response to treatment
- Skin color
- Glasgow Coma Scale (GCS) score

Obstructed Airway, Child/Adult

Treatment

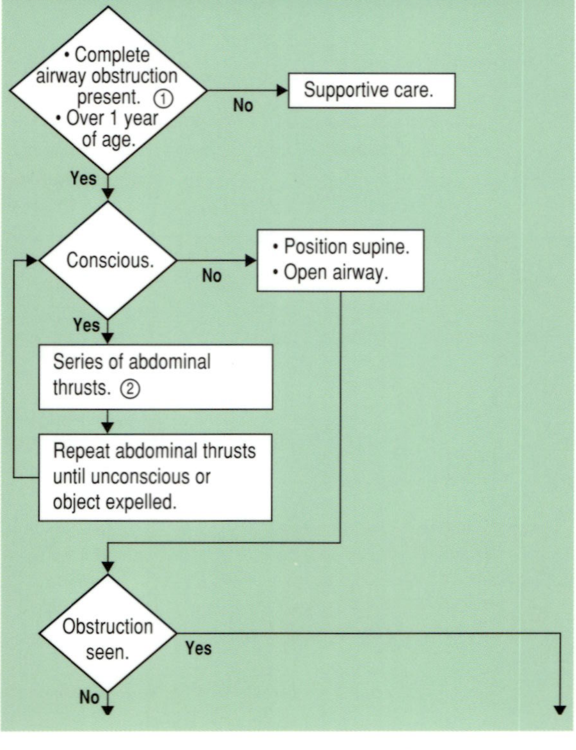

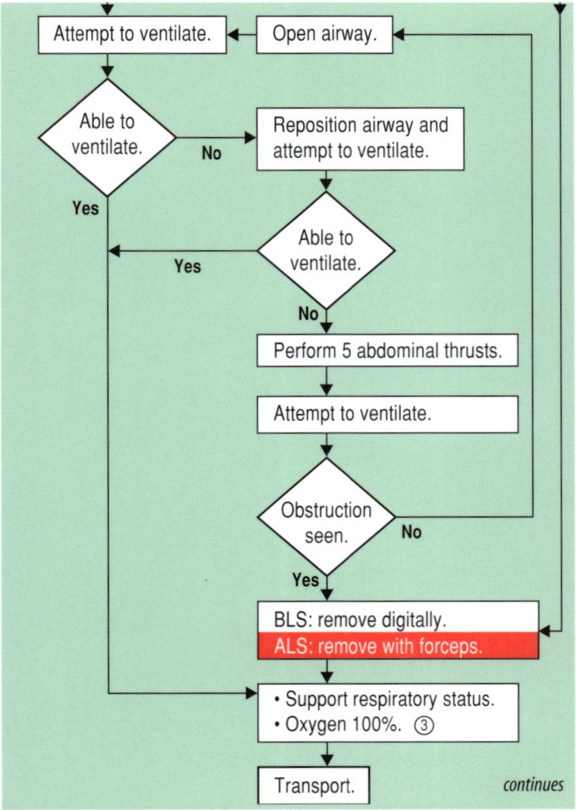

Attempt to ventilate.
Open airway.
Able to ventilate.
No
Yes
Reposition airway and attempt to ventilate.
Able to ventilate.
Yes
No
Perform 5 abdominal thrusts.
Attempt to ventilate.
Obstruction seen.
No
Yes
BLS: remove digitally.
ALS: remove with forceps.
• Support respiratory status.
• Oxygen 100%. ③
Transport.

continues

1. This protocol assumes the patient has a pulse. Assessment: Ask the patient, "Are you choking?"
2. Chest thrusts may be used if the patient is obese or pregnant and the caregiver cannot reach his or her arms around the patient.
3. Assist ventilations until consciousness returns. Consider need for intubation.

Obstructed Airway, Infant

Treatment

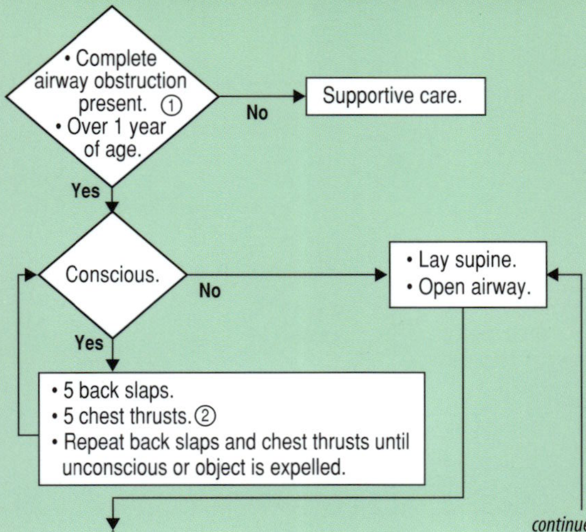

continues

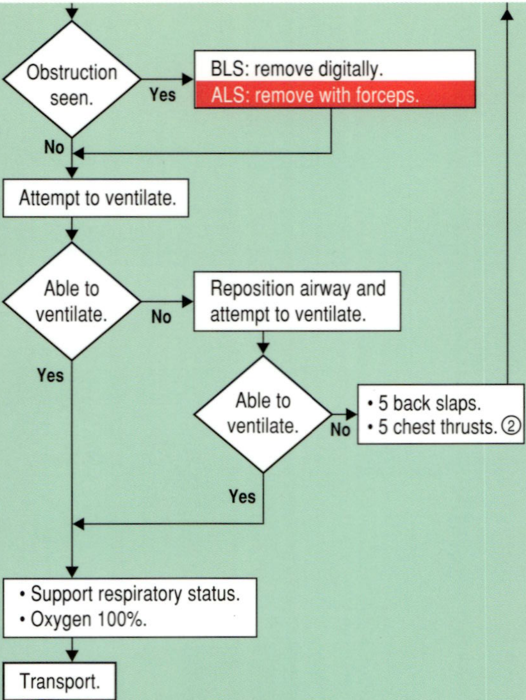

1. This protocol assumes the patient has a pulse.
2. Chest thrusts are slower than chest compressions. Place head lower than trunk.

Amputation

Considerations

If an extremity is involved and venous or arterial bleeding cannot be stopped with direct pressure, a tourniquet should be applied. The tourniquet should be gradually tightened until the bleeding has stopped. Note the time the tourniquet was applied.

Assessment

- Airway, breathing, circulation.
- Administer oxygen via nasal cannula, as needed. If active bleeding is present or if blood loss is significant, administer a higher concentration using a nonrebreathing mask.
- Control bleeding (direct pressure, tourniquet).
- BLS to consider ALS. Transport ASAP. Consider air transport if scene time is delayed.
- Stump: Cover with a moist, sterile dressing, covered by a dry dressing.
- Amputated tissue: Wrap in sterile, moistened gauze and seal in a plastic bag. Place the bag over ice. The tissue should not come into direct contact with the ice or soak in water.

Treatment

- ABCs.
- Oxygen 100%, SpO_2. ①
- Assist ventilations, as needed.
- Consider spinal immobilization.
- Keep patient warm.
- Transport ASAP.

↓

continues

Treatment, continued

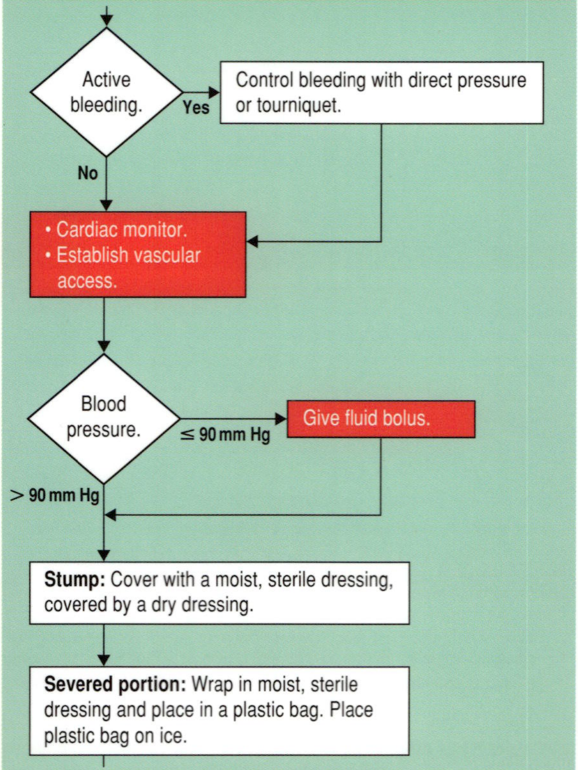

Extreme pain.

Yes → Consider pain management:
Morphine 0.1 mg/kg up to 10 mg.
OR
fentanyl 1 mcg/kg up to 100 mcg.
Titrate slowly. Contact medical command.

No →

- Transport ASAP. ②
- Estimate blood loss.
- Keep patient warm.

1. If active bleeding is present or if blood loss is significant, administer a higher concentration using a nonrebreathing mask.
2. If scene time is delayed or extensive (i.e., lengthy extrication), consider air transport.

Pediatric Considerations

ALS

Morphine: 0.1 mg/kg up to 10 mg. Titrate slowly.

Fentanyl: 1 mcg/kg up to 100 mcg.

Documentation

- Mechanism of injury
- Time of injury
- Time tourniquet applied

Burns

Considerations

- Consider carbon monoxide poisoning.
- Administer 100% high-flow oxygen.
- Transport burn patients to the most appropriate facility.

Palmar Method

The Palmar Method is a mechanism of assessing the total body surface area (BSA) burned. This assessment uses the size of the patient's hand (including the fingers) to represent about 1% of the patient's body surface area.

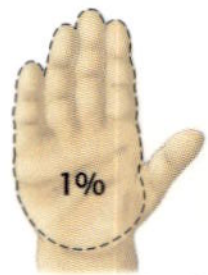

Palmar Method (patient's palm)

The Rule of 9's

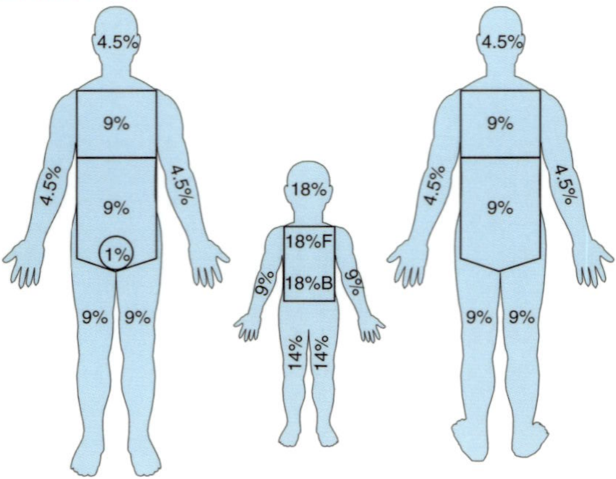

Adult (front) | Infant | Adult (back)

Assessment

- Airway, breathing, circulation.
- If patient is in respiratory distress, apply 100% oxygen. Assist ventilations, as needed.
- Immobilize the spine, if indicated.
- Stop the burning process and prevent unnecessary cooling.
- Focus assessment on depth and extent of burn. The patient's hand represents 1% of his or her body surface area (BSA). Use this as a reference.
- Apply a clean sheet or blankets to prevent hypothermia.
- Transport ASAP.

Stop the Burning Process

- **Thermal:** Remove patient from environment.
- **Tar:** Cool with water or NS. Do not attempt to remove the tar.
- **Chemical:** Brush dry chemicals off. Flush skin with copious amounts of water for 15 to 20 minutes. Avoid getting particles airborne. Do not attempt to neutralize. Consider need for HAZMAT.
- **Electrical:** Make sure the patient is de-energized before approaching. Suspect internal injuries. Look for entrance and exit wounds.

Treatment

- ABCs.
- Oxygen 100%, SpO_2.
- Assist ventilations, as needed.
- Consider spinal immobilization.
- Keep patient warm.
- Transport ASAP. ①

↓

continues

Treatment, continued

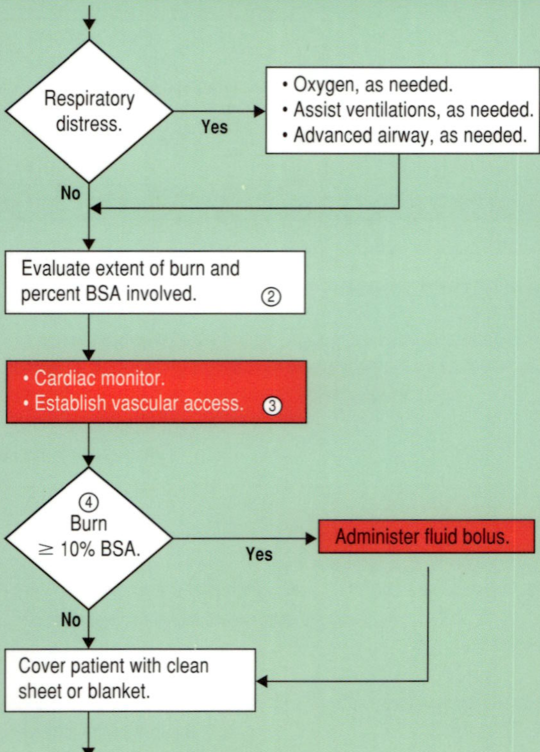

Pain management:
Morphine: 0.1 mg/kg up to 10 mg.
Fentanyl: 1 mcg/kg up to 100 mcg.

- Notify receiving facility ASAP.
- Prevent unnecessary cooling.
- Monitor LOC, vital signs, SpO_2, capnography, respiratory status.

Contact medical command.

Parkland formula:

- The amount of IV fluid the patient will need for the first 24 hours: 4 mL of Lactated Ringer's × the patient's weight (in kg) × the % BSA burned.
- Give half of the total fluid within the first 8 hours of the burn. Give the second half over the next 16 hours.

1. Burns without other trauma, take to burn center; with other trauma, take to trauma center.
2. The patient's hand represents 1% of his or her BSA. Use this as a reference.
3. Start IVs within unburned areas, if possible. Burned areas may be used, if needed.

continues

Treatment, continued

4. American Burn Association transport guidelines for taking patients to burn centers:
   - Partial thickness burn, surface area ≥ to 10% BSA
   - Full-thickness burns
   - Chemical, electrical, or smoke-inhalation burns
   - Burns involving the hands, face, feet, genitalia, or major joints
   - Burns requiring long-term rehabilitation and/or psychological support
   - Patients with pre-existing serious medical history

Pediatric Considerations

ALS

- If trauma is accompanied by burns, substitute NS for Lactated Ringer's (LR) solution.
- Administer a rapid fluid bolus of LR 20 mL/kg via IV/IO or NS 20 mL/kg (if trauma is accompanied by burns).
- Morphine and fentanyl dosages are identical for pediatric and adult patients.

Documentation

- Degree (depth) of burn
- Extent of burn (percent BSA involved)
- Mechanism of injury
- Type of burn (chemical, thermal, electrical, scald, contact, smoke inhalation)
- Respiratory status
- Sign of inhalation (singed nares, soot in mouth)
- Oxygen saturation (SpO_2)
- Entrapment

Eye Injuries

Assessment

- Airway, breathing, circulation.
- Impaled object: Do not remove. Dress affected eye and secure object.
- Chemical burn: Flush affected eye with normal saline.
- Offer orientation and reassurance.
- Calculate Glasgow Coma Scale (GCS) score.
- Calculate Revised Trauma Score (RTS).
- Transport.

Treatment

- ABCs.
- Oxygen 100%, SpO_2.
- Assist ventilations, as needed.
- Consider spinal immobilization.
- Keep patient warm.
- Transport ASAP.

Impaled object.

- Yes → Do not remove. → Dress affected eyes and secure object.
- No →

continues

Treatment, continued

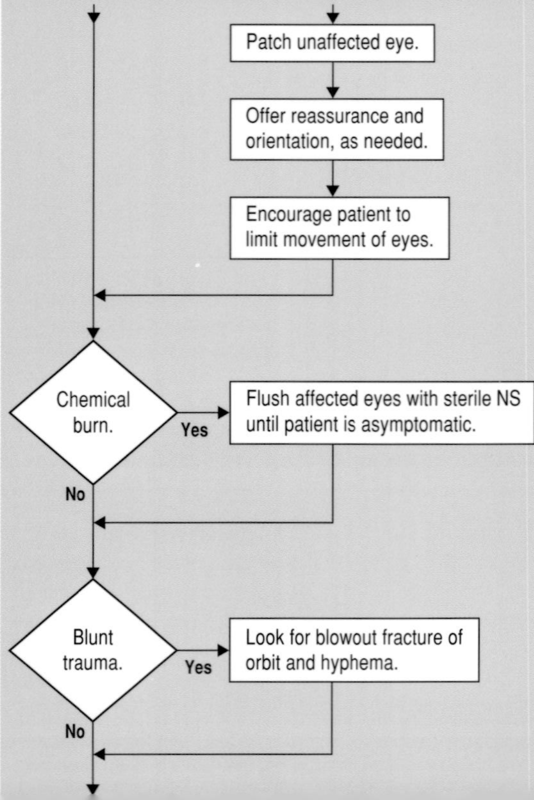

Contact medical command if a problem or question arises.

Documentation

- Signs and symptoms
- Appearance of eye: **P**upils **E**qual **A**nd **R**ound, **R**egular in size, react to **L**ight (PEARRL)
- Cardiac rhythm, if obtained
- Mechanism of injury
- Intensity and duration of pain
- Vital signs
- Oxygen saturation (SpO_2)
- Treatment
- Response to treatment
- GCS score
- Revised Trauma Score (RTS)

General Management of Trauma

Considerations

Patients can be transported by ground or air. The goal is to get the patient to the emergency department in the least possible amount of time. Refer to pages 32 and 33 of this Field Guide for air transport considerations.

Assessment

- Airway, breathing, circulation.
- Consider spinal immobilization.
- Administer 100% oxygen via nonrebreathing mask.
- Assist ventilations, as needed.
- Calculate Glasgow Coma Scale (GCS) score.
- Calculate Revised Trauma Score (RTS).
- Control external bleeding.
- BLS to consider ALS (advanced airway, IV fluids).
- Transport ASAP.

Treatment

- Airway.
- Consider spinal immobilization.
- Transport to appropriate trauma center ASAP. ①
- Limit scene time as much as possible.

↓

Breathing: ②
- Assist ventilations, as needed.
- Oxygen 100%.

↓

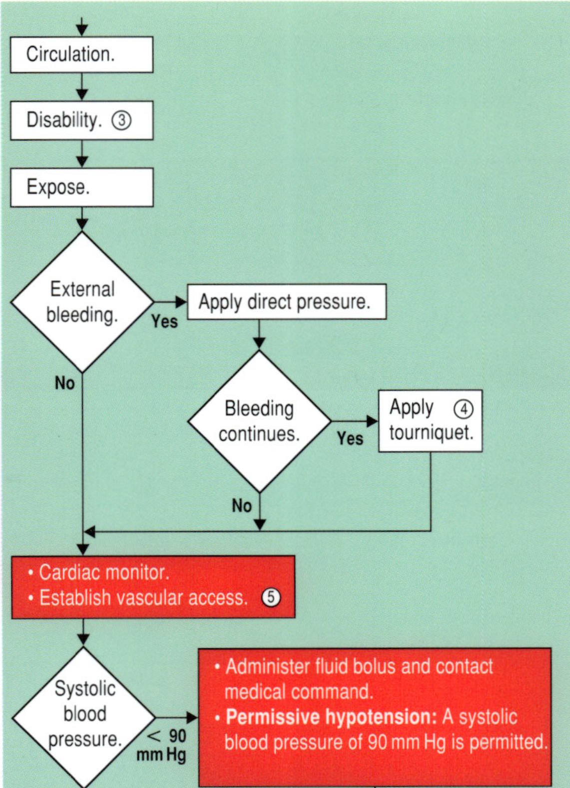

Circulation.
Disability. ③
Expose.
External bleeding.
Yes
Apply direct pressure.
Bleeding continues.
Yes
Apply tourniquet. ④
No
No
• Cardiac monitor.
• Establish vascular access. ⑤
Systolic blood pressure.
< 90 mm Hg
• Administer fluid bolus and contact medical command.
• Permissive hypotension: A systolic blood pressure of 90 mm Hg is permitted.

continues

Treatment, continued

> 90 mm Hg

- Keep patient warm.
- Notify hospital ASAP.

1. Transport in left lateral recumbent position if patient is pregnant.
2. Advanced airway, as needed.
3. Calculate GCS score and Revised Trauma Score (RTS).
4. Apply tourniquet for trauma involving extremities only.
5. Establish two large-bore IV lines of Lactated Ringer's solution or NS. Titrate to maintain systolic blood pressure > 90 mm Hg and a pulse rate < 120 beats/min. Do not delay transport at any time in this protocol.

Pediatric Considerations

ALS

- If trauma is accompanied by burns, substitute NS for Lactated Ringer's (LR) solution.
- Administer a rapid fluid bolus of LR 20 mL/kg via IV/IO or NS 20 mL/kg (if trauma is accompanied by burns).
- Morphine and fentanyl dosages are identical for both pediatric and adult patients.

Documentation

- Signs and symptoms
- GCS score
- Revised Trauma Score (RTS)
- Neurologic status
- Onset and duration of loss of consciousness, if any
- Oxygen saturation (SpO_2)
- Cardiac rhythm
- Mechanism of injury

Head and Spine Injuries

Considerations

Every patient who has had a loss of consciousness should be evaluated at a hospital. Open wounds that expose brain tissue should be covered with saline-soaked gauze.

Assessment

- Airway, breathing, circulation.
- Administer 100% oxygen.
- Assist ventilations, as needed.
- Full-spine immobilization.
- Glasgow Coma Scale (GCS) score.
- Revised Trauma Score (RTS).
- BLS to consider ALS (advanced airway, IV fluids).

Treatment

- ABCs.
- Oxygen 100%, SpO_2.
- Assist ventilations, as needed.
- Consider spinal immobilization.
- Keep patient warm.
- Transport ASAP. ① ②

↓

- Calculate GCS score.
- Assess dermatome level involved.

↓

continues

Treatment, continued

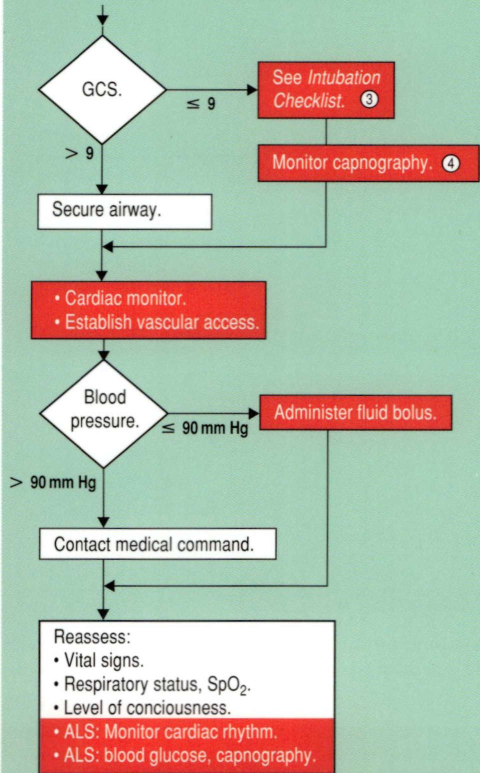

1. Every patient who has had a loss of consciousness should be evaluated at a hospital.
2. Transport in left lateral recumbant position if patient is pregnant.
3. Do not attempt nasal intubation.
4. Maintain end-tidal carbon dioxide between 25 mm Hg and 35 mm Hg.

Documentation

- Signs and symptoms
- GCS score
- Revised Trauma Score (RTS)
- Onset and duration of loss of consciousness
- Oxygen saturation (SpO_2)
- Cardiac rhythm
- Motor function/sensation
- Mechanism of injury

Orthopedic Injuries

Considerations

- Check distal pulses, motor function, and sensation before and after splinting.
- Consider use of pneumatic anti-shock garment (PASG) or pelvic sling to stabilize and splint pelvic fractures.

Assessment

- Airway, breathing, circulation.
- Administer oxygen, as needed.
- Treat life-threatening injuries first.
- Prepare for transport:
  - Immobilize fracture site, splinting above and below the site. If there is significant deformity or if the distal extremity is cyanotic or lacks pulses, align with gentle traction before splinting.
  - Isolated closed femur (mid-shaft) fractures: Apply a traction splint.
  - Pelvic fractures: Consider PASG or a pelvic sling.

Treatment

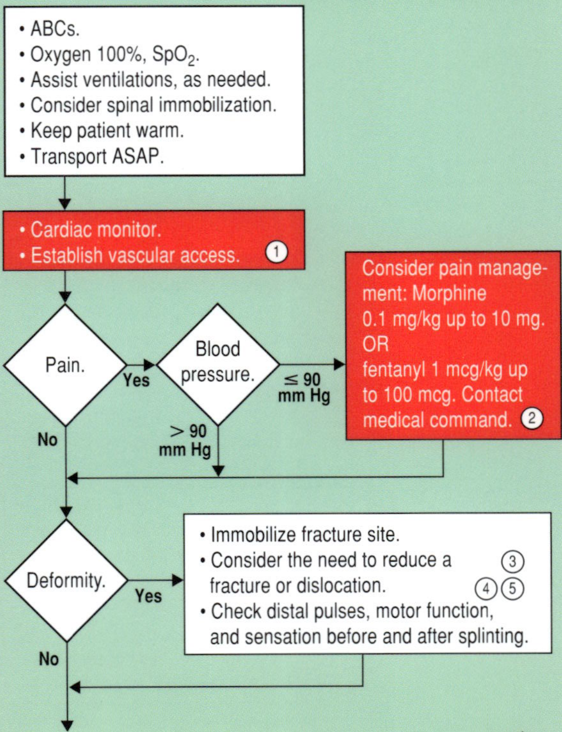

continues

Treatment, continued

↓

- Elevate simple extremity injuries.
- Apply ice to site.

↓

- Keep patient warm.
- Monitor distal pulses, skin temperature, sensation, and motor function.
- Transport ASAP.

1. Start IV NS on any serious injury. Use your judgment on minor fractures.
2. Morphine may cause nausea, especially if given quickly.
3. If there is significant deformity or if the distal extremity is cyanotic or lacks distal pulses, align with gentle traction before splinting.
4. Isolated closed femur (mid-shaft) fractures: Apply a traction splint. Traction splints are contraindicated in the presence of a pelvic, hip, distal femur, and/or lower leg fracture.
5. Pelvic fractures: Consider PASG or a pelvic sling.

Pediatric Considerations

ALS

- If trauma is accompanied by burns, substitute NS for Lactated Ringer's (LR) solution.
- Administer a rapid fluid bolus of LR 20 mL/kg via IV/IO or NS 20 mL/kg (if trauma is accompanied by burns).
- Morphine and fentanyl dosages are identical for pediatric and adult patients.

Documentation

- Signs and symptoms
- Presence and degree of deformity
- Distal circulation
- Motor function
- Sensation
- Oxygen saturation (SpO_2)
- Skin color
- Mechanism of injury

Soft Tissue Injuries

Considerations

Controlling External Bleeding

Direct Pressure: Use a sterile dressing and gloved hand to apply direct, steady pressure over a bleeding site. Maintain the pressure and secure with a roller bandage. If bleeding continues, leave the original dressing in place and apply a second bandage. Elevating the site, if possible, will slow venous bleeding.

Tourniquet: Apply a commercially available tourniquet per manufacturer's instructions. If not available, use wide material, such as a cravat. A blood pressure cuff works well for upper extremities. Wrap the material around the extremity twice at a point approximately 8 cm distal to the axilla or groin and tie a half knot. Place a stick or similar object on top of the half knot, and complete the square knot above the stick. Twist the stick to tighten the tourniquet until the bleeding stops. Secure the stick in that position. Write "TK" and the time you applied the tourniquet on adhesive tape and apply the tape to the patient's forehead. Do not remove the tourniquet.

Management of Specific Injuries

Amputation: Preserve the amputated tissue. Rinse the tissue of debris and wrap it loosely in saline-moistened gauze. Seal tissue in a plastic bag and place in a cool container. Keep the tissue cold, but do not allow it to freeze and do not allow it to soak in water. Transport as quickly as possible. If any delays are expected, consider air transport.

Impaled Object: Do not remove an impaled object unless it interferes with the airway. Stabilize the object in place with a bulky dressing and immobilize the site, if possible. The goal is to limit motion of the impaled object.

Crush Syndrome: Make every effort to treat the patient: start multiple IVs, give IV normal saline (NS) before removing the crushing object. The concern is that the patient will experience severe hypotension and a release of potassium (hyperkalemia). Avoid Lactated Ringer's (LR), because LR has potassium. Contact medical command for direction.

Assessment

- Airway, breathing, circulation.
- Spinal immobilization, as needed.
- Administer 100% oxygen.
- Control external bleeding. See *Considerations*.
- Apply cold compresses for pain.
- Transport ASAP.

Treatment

- ABCs.
- Oxygen 100%, SpO_2.
- Assist ventilations, as needed.
- Consider spinal immobilization.
- Keep patient warm.
- Transport ASAP.

↓

Control external bleeding: Direct pressure and tourniquets may be used to control bleeding. (1)

↓

Apply cold compresses.

↓

- Cardiac monitor.
- Establish vascular access.

↓

continues

Treatment, continued

Consider pain management: Morphine 0.1 mg/kg up to 10 mg. (2)
OR
fentanyl 1 mcg/kg up to 100 mcg. Contact medical command.

- Monitor distal pulses, skin temperature, sensation, and motor function.
- Transport ASAP.

1. Apply tourniquet for extremities only.
2. Morphine may cause nausea, especially if given quickly.

Pediatric Considerations

ALS

- If trauma is accompanied by burns, substitute NS for Lactated Ringer's (LR) solution.
- Administer a rapid fluid bolus of LR 20 mL/kg via IV/IO or NS 20 mL/kg (if trauma is accompanied by burns).
- Morphine and fentanyl dosages are identical for pediatric and adult patients.

Documentation

- Signs and symptoms
- Time tourniquet applied
- Distal neurovascular status: pulse, motor function, sensation
- Oxygen saturation (SpO_2)
- Skin color
- Mechanism of injury

Trauma Transport Guidelines

Considerations

- Steps 1 and 2 of this algorithm attempt to identify the most seriously injured patients. These patients should be transported to the highest level of care within the trauma system.
- See pages 32 and 33 of this Field Guide for air transport considerations.

Treatment

Step 1: Measure vital signs and level of consciousness. Are ANY of the following indicators present?

- GCS: < 14
- Systolic blood pressure: < 90 mm Hg
- Respiratory rate: < 10 or > 29 breaths/min (< 20 breaths/min in infant)

Yes → Take to a trauma center. ①

No → Assess anatomy of injury. ↓

Step 2:

- All penetrating injuries to head, neck, torso, and extremity proximal to elbow and knee
- Flail chest
- Two or more proximal, long-bone fractures
- Crushed, degloved, or mangled extremity
- Amputation proximal to wrist and ankle
- Pelvic fractures
- Open or depressed skull fractures
- Paralysis

Yes → Take to a trauma center. (1)

No → Assess mechanism of injury and evidence of high-energy impact.

Step 3: Falls

- Adults: > 20 feet (one story is equal to ten feet)
- Children: > 10 feet or two to three times their height

High-energy motor vehicle collision

- Intrusion on occupant site 12–18 inches on any side
- Ejection (partial or complete) from automobile
- Death in same passenger compartment
- Vehicle telemetry data consistent with high risk of injury

Auto vs pedestrian/bicyclist: > 20 mph impact

Motorcycle crash: > 20 mph

Yes ↓ **No** ↓

continues

Treatment, continued

Take to closest appropriate trauma center. ②

Assess special patient or system considerations.

Step 4:

- **Age**
  - Older Adults: Risk of death increases after age 55.
  - All NJ trauma centers have pediatric capability.
- **Anticoagulation and bleeding disorders**
- Burns (without other trauma, take to burn center; with other trauma, take to trauma center)
- **Time-sensitive extremity injury**
- **End-stage renal disease** (requiring dialysis)
- **Pregnancy** $>$ 20 weeks
- **EMS provider judgment**

Yes

- Contact medical command.
- Consider transport to a trauma center.

No

Transport according to protocol.

When in doubt, transport to a trauma center.

Adapted from www.cdc.gov/FieldTriage

1. These patients should be taken to the highest level of care within the trauma system.
2. Transport to the closest appropriate trauma center, which, depending on the trauma system, need not be the highest-level trauma center.

Documentation

- Communication with medical command
- Mechanism of injury
- Trauma criteria/indicator
- Activation of trauma system

Cricothyrotomy

Considerations

- Indications: Severe facial or nasal injuries, anaphylaxis, chemical inhalation injury, or when other means of establishing an airway are not adequate.
- Contraindications: Patients whose airway can be secured by an alternate advanced airway.
- Procedure cannot be initiated without approval from medical command.

Assessment

- Airway, breathing, circulation.
- Administer 100% oxygen.
- BLS to request ALS.
- Transport ASAP.

Treatment

Items needed:

- Scalpel
- IV needle/catheter, 10–12 gauge
- Antiseptic solution
- Sterile gloves
- Sterile 4 × 4 gauze pads
- Oxygen
- Bag-valve device
- 3-mm ET tube adapter
- Eye protection
- Jet ventilation tubing

Select site.

↓

Cricothyroid membrane: soft aspect just below the larynx, midline, anterior trachea.

↓

Cleanse site with antiseptic.

Technique

↓

Stabilize larynx between thumb and index finger of nondominant hand.

↓

Palpate cricothyroid membrane.

↓

Using a scalpel, make a 2- to 3-cm vertical incision through the skin over the cricothyroid membrane.

↓

Dab the incision dry with sterile 4 × 4 gauze pads to control capillary oozing.

↓

continues

Treatment, continued

↓

Insert needle (with attached syringe) through the midline of the membrane at a 45° to 60° angle toward the patient's chest, applying negative pressure to the syringe.

↓

Air will enter the syringe when the needle is in the trachea.

↓

Advance the catheter over the needle toward the carina; remove needle and syringe.

↓

Attach a 3-mm ET tube adapter to the hub of the needle. (1)

↓

Hold the catheter in place as you attach bag-valve device to the ET tube adapter.

↓

Ventilate with bag-valve device 100% oxygen.

↓

Confirm successful cannulation: Auscultate breath sounds, monitor SpO_2 and/or end-tidal carbon dioxide, observe chest rise. ②

1. Transtracheal jet ventilation: Optimal ventilation may be achieved by transtracheal jet ventilation. Deliver ventilations at a ratio of 1:4 (1 second of oxygen/jet ventilation, 4 seconds off) to allow passive exhalation. Tubing should be prepared in advance and attached to an oxygen source.
2. If the catheter becomes occluded, irrigate it with 2–3 mL of sterile NS.

Documentation

- Need for cricothyrotomy
- Signs and symptoms
- Procedure/technique
- Treatment
- Response to treatment
- Oxygen saturation (SpO_2)
- End-tidal carbon dioxide

Epinephrine Auto-Injector

This procedure applies to NJDHSS registered epinephrine auto-injector agencies only.

Considerations

1. If the patient has his or her own prescribed epinephrine auto-injector and it is immediately available, use it.
2. If credible history determines that the patient has been given an appropriate dose of epinephrine prior to your arrival, allow at least 10 minutes from the reported time of injection for symptoms to improve. Reevaluate vital signs and clinical status.
3. Use appropriate epinephrine auto-injector from your vehicle stock as additional dose (if needed) after use of patient's own auto-injector or as only dose if patient does not have one.
4. Clinical criteria to administer is the same, regardless of whether the auto-injector is carried by EMS or it belongs to the patient.
5. Verbal notification shall be made to the Office of Emergency Medical Services (OEMS) within 72 hours of administration by the EMT or the BLS agency. Copies of the patient care report shall be mailed to the OEMS within 45 days of administration. BLS agencies must register with the OEMS to carry epinephrine auto-injectors.

Assessment

- Airway, breathing, circulation.
- Administer 100% oxygen via nonrebreathing (NRB) mask at a rate of 15 L/min. If unable to tolerate mask, administer via nasal cannula at a rate of 1–6 L/min.
- BLS to request ALS.
- Obtain vital signs and SAMPLE history.
- Initiate treatment with the appropriate epinephrine auto-injector if anaphylaxis is present. Look for the following indications of anaphylaxis: respiratory distress or arrest; a tight feeling in the chest or throat; wheezing; stridor; restlessness; confusion; unconsciousness; seizure; generalized urticaria; swelling of the face, tongue, or lips; and hypoperfusion with increased heart rate:

  - **Age 0–12 months:** pulse > 180 beats/min and/or systolic blood pressure < 60 mm Hg
  - **Age 1–12 years:** pulse > 140 beats/min and/or systolic blood pressure < 70 mm Hg
  - **Older than 12 years:** pulse > 120 beats/min and/or systolic blood pressure < 80 mm Hg
- Transport ASAP.

Epinephrine Administration

Dose amount: Younger than 4 years, use the auto-injector that delivers 0.15 mg; 4 years and older, use the auto-injector that delivers 0.3 mg.

1. Check the medication.
2. Remove the auto-injector safety cap.
3. Place the auto-injector against the lateral portion of the patient's thigh, midway between the waist and the knee.
4. Push auto-injector firmly against site until injector activates.
5. Hold the auto-injector in place for 10 seconds to make sure the medication is injected.
6. Using a straight motion, pull the injector from the injection site.
7. Dispose of the auto-injector into a biohazard container.
8. Record the location of the injection site, time, dose, medication, vital signs, and changes in patient condition.
9. Continuously monitor the patient. Maintain normal body temperature.
10. Contact medical command if problem or question arises.

Documentation

- Location of the injection site
- Time
- Dose
- Medication
- Vital signs
- Changes in patient condition
- Signs and symptoms
- Cardiac rhythm, if obtained
- Oxygen saturation (SpO_2)
- Response to treatment

Intraosseous Infusion

Considerations

- Technique varies based on the type of supplies and equipment used. Follow the manufacturer's guidelines.
- Indications: Urgent need to administer IV fluid or medications.
- Contraindications: Trauma at proposed site, infection at proposed site.

Assessment

- Airway, breathing, circulation.
- BLS to request ALS.
- Transport ASAP.

Treatment

Select site.

↓

- Proximal tibia: anterior-medial aspect, 2–3 cm below the tibial tuberosity.
- Proximal humerus.
- Sternum. ①

Prepare site.

↓

Restrain, secure extremity.

↓

Prep site with antiseptic.

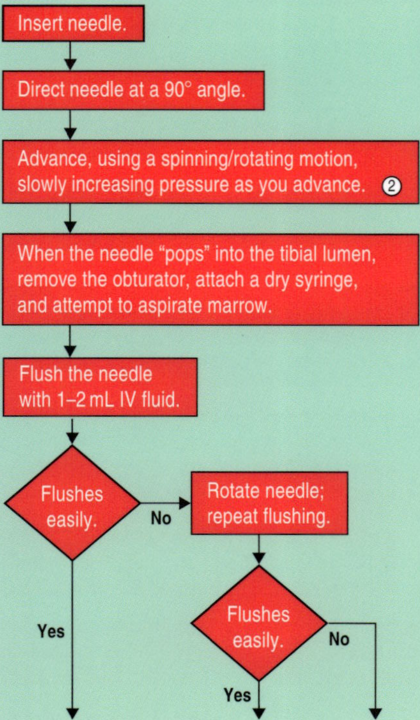
Insert needle.
Direct needle at a 90° angle.
Advance, using a spinning/rotating motion, slowly increasing pressure as you advance. ②
When the needle "pops" into the tibial lumen, remove the obturator, attach a dry syringe, and attempt to aspirate marrow.
Flush the needle with 1–2 mL IV fluid.
Flushes easily.
No
Rotate needle; repeat flushing.
Flushes easily.
Yes
No
Yes

continues

Treatment, continued

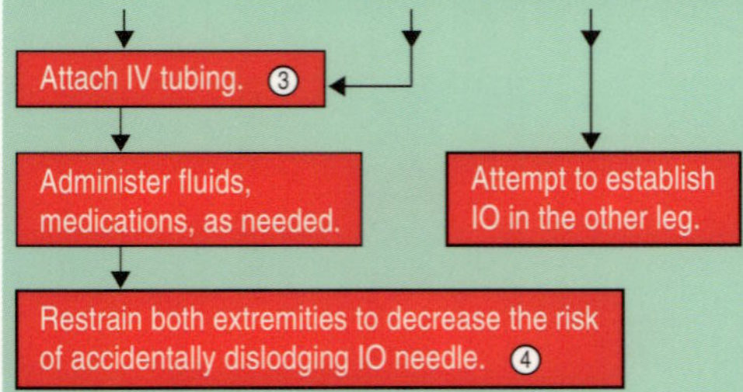

1. Follow the manufacturer's recommendations regarding site selection and proper approach to that site.
2. Avoid using a rocking motion.
3. Use a three-way stopcock and a 60-mL syringe to administer fluid via boluses.
4. Children will often move the unaffected leg and accidentally dislodge the IO needle. Secure both legs as soon as possible. Contact medical command.

Documentation

- Insertion site
- Signs and symptoms
- Time of IV/IO therapy
- Time of contact with medical command

Intubation Checklist

Considerations

- Keep the patient warm. Paralyzed patients lose their ability to generate body heat.
- Creating a sniffing position where the patient's earlobe and sternal notch are level with each other is ideal and will bring all of the intubation angles into place. Do not move the patient's neck into an exaggerated sniffing position if c-spine precautions are in place.
- When properly performed, cricoid pressure applies pressure to the inferior aspect of the larynx (thyroid cartilage).
- These procedures shall not delay the transport of a patient in the event of a difficult intubation. Advanced interventions shall only be attempted after all BLS interventions have been instituted.

Assessment (BLS Assisting ALS with Intubation)

- Airway, breathing, circulation.
- Administer 100% oxygen via bag-mask.
- Obtain history. Does the patient have allergies?

Difficult airway: Consider alternative advanced airway prior to intubation.

Preparation

- [ ] Rule out allergies.
- [ ] Pre-oxygenate 100% oxygen per BVM.
- [ ] SpO_2 probe on and reading.

continues

- [ ] Suction on, Yankauer tip in place.
- [ ] Consider other advanced airways.
- [ ] Extra ETTs: one larger, one smaller.
- [ ] Bougie, end-tidal CO_2 detector at hand.
- [ ] Stethoscope, multiple blades at hand.
- [ ] Alternative airway at hand.

Patient (procedure)

- [ ] Examine patient, difficult airway?
- [ ] Earlobe level with sternal notch. ①
- [ ] Consider cricoid pressure. ②
- [ ] Rapid sequence intubation (RSI): Approved for age 13 or older.
  - [ ] If head injury present: lidocaine 1 mg/kg IV
  - [ ] Atropine: 0.01 mg/kg

- ☐ Midazolam (Versed): 0.1 mg/kg normal BP ③ OR etomidate (Amidate): 0.3 mg/kg low BP
- ☐ Succinylcholine (Anectine): 1.5 mg/kg ④
- ☐ Rocuronium (Zemuron): 0.6–1.2 mg/kg
- ☐ Vecuronium (Norcuron): 0.1 mg/kg
- ☐ Ketamine: 0.2–1 mg/kg IV

Post-Intubation

- ☐ Confirm ETT placement.
- ☐ Secure ET tube with commercial device.
- ☐ Continued sedation/paralysis:
  - ☐ Midazolam (Versed): 0.1 mg/kg IV if BP normal or elevated
  - ☐ Ativan (Lorazepam): 0.5–2 mg/kg
  - ☐ Vecuronium (Norcuron): 0.1 mg/kg IV

continues

1. To obtain the appropriate sniffing position, elevate the patient's head so that the patient's earlobe is level or even with the patient's sternal notch. Do NOT move the patient's neck if possibility of c-spine injury exists.
2. Cricoid pressure: When performed properly, the caregiver is applying pressure to the inferior aspect of the larynx (thyroid cartilage).
3. Consider pain-control measures. Neither paralytics nor sedatives provide pain control.
4. Succinylcholine (Anectine): Obtain history. Do not give succinylcholine (Anectine) if familial history of malignant hyperthermia is noted. Succinylcholine (Anectine) is contraindicated in penetrating eye injury, in severe burns or crush injuries that are 2 to 5 days old, in the presence of hyperkalemia, and in patients with chronic muscular conditions (i.e., muscular dystrophy). The onset of succinylcholine (Anectine) is 30–60 seconds; duration is 8–10 minutes.

Documentation

- Airway
- Respiratory status
- Oxygen saturation (SpO_2)
- End-tidal carbon dioxide
- Endotracheal tube (ETT) size/length (cm at the patient's teeth)
- Confirmation of ETT placement (mist in the ETT, end-tidal carbon dioxide color change, bilateral lung sounds, chest rise, skin color)

Oxygen Administration

Hypoxic drive: A healthy patient exhales because the body detects the presence of carbon dioxide. Some patients with chronic obstructive pulmonary disease (COPD), unlike a healthy patient, use their hypoxic drive (exhale/inhale because their body detects lower oxygen level). When COPD patients who are using their hypoxic drive are given too much oxygen, their respiratory drive may decrease or stop when their body detects ample oxygen. As a result, expect and accept oxygen saturation (SpO_2) readings below 90% and above 85% on patients with COPD. Give lower concentrations (2–3 L/min via nasal cannula) to these patients, **but never deprive a patient in respiratory distress of oxygen. If a patient is in respiratory distress, give high concentrations of oxygen.**

Table 1 outlines oxygen delivery devices, their flow rates, and the percentage of oxygen delivered.

TABLE 1 Oxygen Delivery Devices

Device	Flow Rate	Oxygen Delivered
Bag-mask device with reservoir	15 L/min	Nearly 100%
CPAP	15 to 25 L/min	Nearly 100%
Mouth-to-mask device	15 L/min	Nearly 55%
Nasal cannula (NC)	1 to 6 L/min	24% to 44%
Nonrebreathing mask (NRB)	10 to 15 L/min	Up to 90%
Venturi mask	12 to 15 L/min	24% to 60%

ST-Segment Elevation Myocardial Infarction (STEMI)

Considerations

Consider atypical presentation (vague complaints) in female, diabetic, or elderly patients and for patients with return of spontaneous circulation (ROSC) post cardiac arrest.

Assessment

- Airway, breathing, circulation.
- Oxygen 100%.
- BLS to request ALS when the patient presents with signs and symptoms of acute coronary syndrome (chest pain or pressure, shortness of breath, nausea, diaphoresis).
- Place the patient in a position of comfort.
- **BLS: Nitroglycerin administration:** You may assist the patient to administer nitroglycerin 0.4 mg if:
  - The patient possesses his or her own prescribed nitroglycerin in either tablet or spray form (0.4 mg per dose),
  - AND the patient's systolic blood pressure is equal to or greater than 100 mm Hg,
  - AND the patient has NOT taken the maximum of three doses within the past 15 minutes.
- Nitroglycerin is contraindicated if the patient is taking Viagra, Levitra, Cialis, or another erectile dysfunction medication.
- Monitor relief of discomfort after interventions using a pain scale of 1 to 10.
- **BLS: Aspirin administration:** You may assist the patient with administration of aspirin* up to 325 mg if:
  - The patient is at least 19 years old,
  - AND the patient has NOT taken the maximum 325 mg dose for this episode.

* Have patient chew then swallow the aspirin (even if not a "chewable" tablet).

Treatment

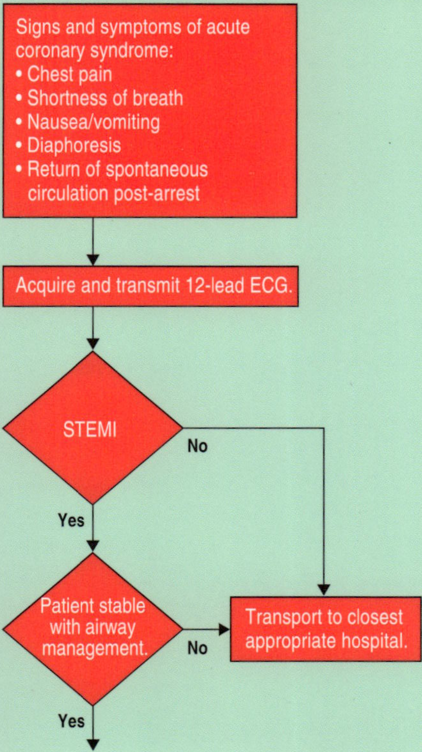

continues

Treatment, continued

↓

Transport to PCI center.

↓

Alert PCI center.

Documentation

- Signs and symptoms
- Electrocardiogram (ECG)
- Cardiac rhythm
- Nature, intensity, and duration of pain
- Vital signs
- Oxygen saturation (SpO_2)
- Treatment
- Response to treatment
- Consultation with medical command

Act F.A.S.T. Stroke Assessment

Assessment

BLS

- Support ABCs; provide oxygen.
- Perform Act F.A.S.T. stroke assessment.
- Establish time when patient was known normal.
- Obtain witness/contact name and cell number.
- Transport to Stroke Center if stable.
- Alert Stroke Center.

ALS

- Initiate vascular access.
- Check blood glucose.
- Obtain electrocardiogram (ECG).
- Contact medical command.
- Do not treat hypertension.

The acronym F.A.S.T. teaches the signs and symptoms of stroke. The acronym stands for:

F Face: Ask the patient to smile. Is there facial droop? Are there drooping eyelids?

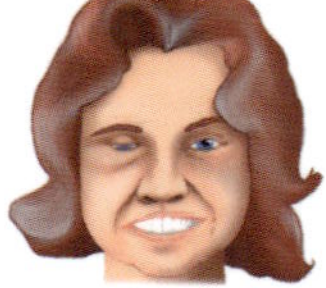

continues

A Arms: Ask the patient to extend his or her arms. Is one arm drifting downward, turning toward the body?

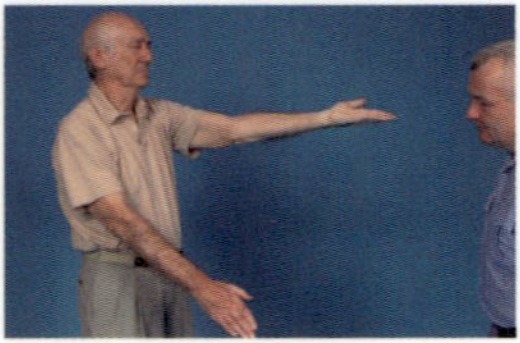

S Speech: Ask the patient to speak. Is the speech slurred? Are the words appropriate?

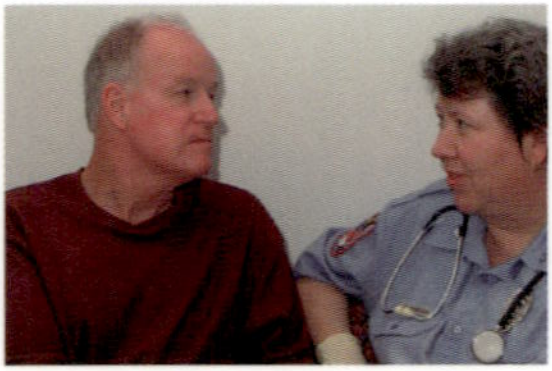

T Time: If the patient is showing these symptoms, time is important! Transport ASAP.

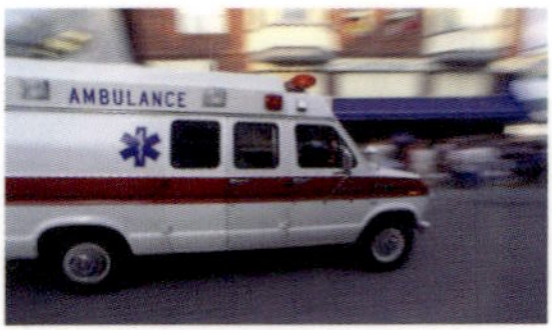

Tension Pneumothorax Decompression

Considerations

Signs and symptoms of tension pneumothorax include, shock, respiratory distress, decreased breath sounds on the affected side, jugular vein distention, increased resistance to positive ventilation, tracheal deviation, and asymmetrical chest rise.

Assessment

- Airway, breathing, circulation.
- Administer 100% oxygen, as needed.
- Assist ventilations, as needed.
- BLS to request ALS.
- Transport ASAP.

Treatment

- ABCs.
- Oxygen 100%.
- Assist ventilations, as needed.
- Transport ASAP.

Items needed:

- IV needle/catheter: 10- to 14-gauge or device specifically designed to decompress a pneumothorax
- Antiseptic solution
- 5–10 mL syringe
- One-way valve
- Tape
- Sterile gloves if available

Select site to decompress: affected side, second intercostal space, midclavicular line.

continues

Treatment, continued

↓

Cleanse site with antiseptic.

↓

Insert 10- to 14-gauge needle. Advance over the superior aspect of the third rib. Attempt to aspirate with an attached syringe as you advance. (1)

↓

If under tension, air may fill the syringe.

↓

If blood is aspirated, consider hemothorax.

↓

Advance catheter and remove needle and syringe.

↓

Attach one-way valve and secure to patient's chest.

↓

Auscultate breath sounds frequently.

↓

Monitor SpO_2, cardiac rhythm, clinical status, and, if intubated, end-tidal carbon dioxide.

1. As an option, you can add 2–3 mL sterile NS to the syringe. If the lung is decompressed, air may bubble into the syringe, giving you a visual clue that air is escaping the chest during insertion.

Documentation

- Respiratory effort and lung sounds before and after procedure
- Site selection
- Oxygen saturation (SpO_2)

Ventricular Assist Devices (VADs)

911 Called

Always attempt to:
- Request ALS if appropriate
- Contact VAD Implant Center
- Keep patient's companion/family member with the patient
- Bring VAD equipment with you
- Transport to VAD Implant Center
- Consider air medical transport

Patient Problem
- Volume related (bleeding/ infection)
- Arrhythmia
- Heart failure
- Non-cardiac related emergency

Patient Stable

Signs of good perfusion: (alert, oriented, good skin color/temperature)
- Contact VAD Center
- Treat per recommendations or standard protocol
- Transport urgently to ED or VAD Center

Pump Problem
- Battery/power
- Controller related
- Internal device related

CONTACT VAD CENTER

Battery/Power
- Replace battery
- Attach to wall outlet

DO NOT RESTART UNLESS INSTRUCTED TO DO SO BY VAD CENTER

Controller Related
- Switch to spare controller

Patient Unstable

Signs of poor perfusion: (altered mental status, cyanosis, cool skin, unresponsive)

- Treat with standard protocol
- Consider fluid bolus
- OK to administer medications
- OK to use electrical therapy
- Transport urgently to ED or VAD Center
- AVOID CHEST COMPRESSIONS

Internal Device Related

- Support circulation

VAD Patient Facts

- Patient may or may not have a palpable pulse normally.
- Blood pressure is normally audible by doppler only.
- Most patients wear a MedicAlert tag showing the VAD Center contact information.
- Controller alarm colors same as triage colors (Red: Urgent, Yellow: Emergent, Green: Time to take action).
- Be careful with scissors—lots of wires and tubing.

NJ VAD Centers—Emergency Phone Numbers

Make every effort to speak with VAD Coordinator or On-call Team

Hackensack University Medical Center:	201-996-4849
Newark Beth Israel Medical Center:	973-926-7205
Morristown Memorial Hospital:	973-971-4179
RWJ—University Hospital:	732-253-3699

Emergency Preparedness Definitions

Control zones Areas at an incident that are designated as hot, warm, or cold, based on safety issues and the degree of hazard found there.

Hazardous materials (HAZMAT) Any substance or material that is capable of posing an unreasonable risk to human health, safety, or the environment when transported in commerce, used incorrectly, or not properly contained or stored.

Incident commander (IC) The overall leader of the incident command system.

Incident command system (ICS) A system implemented to manage disasters and mass casualty incidents in which section chiefs, including finance, logistics, operations, and planning, report to the incident commander.

Joint Information System (JIS) A system that ensures coordination and information accuracy between response agencies.

Mass casualty incident (MCI) An event in which the number of patients exceeds the available resources in the initial response.

Personal protective equipment (PPE) Clothing and gear designed to create a barrier against workplace hazards, as well as to prevent injury from incorrect use or malfunction of equipment.

Regional Operations and Intelligence Center (ROIC) The New Jersey state command center that serves as the foundation for the state's homeland security, crime fighting, and emergency response efforts.

Terrorism The use or violence against persons or property in violation of the criminal laws of the United States for purposes of intimidation, coercion, or ransom.

Triage "Sorting" your patients based on the severity of their injuries. There are five common triage categories: Immediate (red tag), Delayed (yellow tag), Minor (green tag), Deceased (black tag), and Uninjured (white tag).

Unified command An incident command option that allows representatives from multiple jurisdictions and/or agencies to share command authority and responsibility, working together as a "joint" incident command team.

Weapons of mass destruction (WMD) Any agent designed to bring about mass death, casualties, and/or massive damage to property and infrastructure (bridges, tunnels, airports, and seaports).

EMS Task Force

Mission

- To provide New Jersey and the region with specialized, modular component EMS resources to support operations at major incidents and preplanned events throughout the state's Emergency Management System
- To focus on CBRNE preparation and response and to provide specialized EMS and other resources
- To not take the place of existing mutual aid procedures and command structures
- To be NIMS compliant

Background

- The Task Force supports the Urban Area Security Initiative (UASI) region in New Jersey.
- The UASI region is most vulnerable in New Jersey due to:
  - Greatest infrastructure
  - Highest vulnerabilities and risk
  - Population density
  - Proximity to New York City (#1 target)

Structure of the Task Force

- Consists of EMTs, paramedics, nurses, physicians, and others who will specialize in any one (or more) of the following areas of specialization:

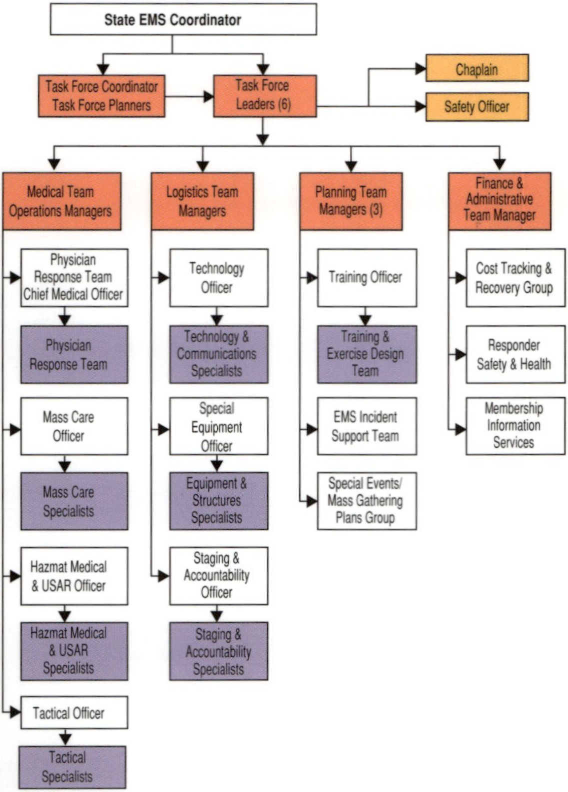

State EMS Coordinator
Task Force Coordinator
Task Force Planners
Task Force Leaders (6)
Chaplain
Safety Officer
Medical Team Operations Managers
Logistics Team Managers
Planning Team Managers (3)
Finance & Administrative Team Manager
Physician Response Team Chief Medical Officer
Physician Response Team
Mass Care Officer
Mass Care Specialists
Hazmat Medical & USAR Officer
Hazmat Medical & USAR Specialists
Tactical Officer
Tactical Specialists
Technology Officer
Technology & Communications Specialists
Special Equipment Officer
Equipment & Structures Specialists
Staging & Accountability Officer
Staging & Accountability Specialists
Training Officer
Training & Exercise Design Team
EMS Incident Support Team
Special Events/ Mass Gathering Plans Group
Cost Tracking & Recovery Group
Responder Safety & Health
Membership Information Services

- Designed to be deployed in modules that are activated based on the needs of an event.
- Many modules are operational and some are still under development.
- Specialized operational modules include:
  - Incident Advanced Team
  - EMS HAZMAT Team
  - Medical Operations Team
  - Logistics Team
  - Staging and Accountability Team
  - Helibase Management Team
  - Communications and Technology Team
  - Safety Team

Activation

New Jersey EMS Task Force assets are requested through the County OEM-EMS Coordinator when county/regional mutual aid resources are insufficient to support an incident.

Communication Centers

Primary Center: REMCS

- Single point of contact to ensure coordination
- Emergency lines: **(973) 972-0911** or **(973) 973-7000**
- Nonemergency lines: **(800) 631-3444** or **(973) 972-6290**
- Emergency Air Medical Requests: **(800) 332-HELO (4356)**

Secondary Center: MEDCENTRAL

- Robert Wood Johnson University Hospital Emergency Medical Services MEDCENTRAL is the designated backup communications center:
  - Emergency line: **(800) 660-1148**
  - Nonemergency line: **(732) 937-8687**

Contact Information

State EMS Coordinator

(609) 633-7777 (Office)

Task Force Coordinator

(609) 633-7777 (Office)

Hazardous Materials

BLS Response

Approaching the Scene

- Approach cautiously from upwind and uphill.
- Position vehicle well away from the incident and facing away from the scene.
- If you are the first on the scene, establish incident command until the HAZMAT team arrives.
- Confirm that the HAZMAT team and fire department have been notified.
- Isolate the scene.
- Keep others away.

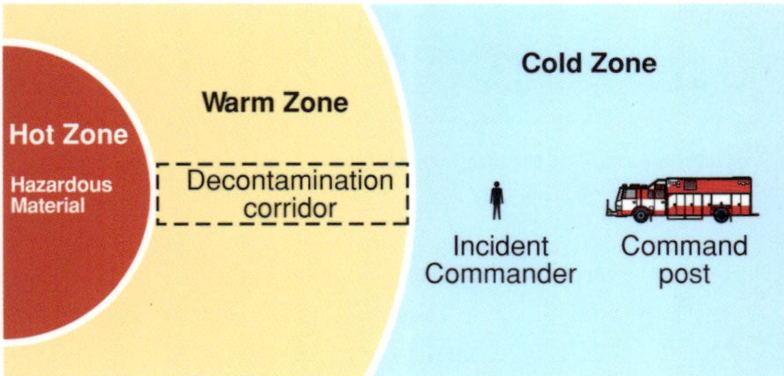

Patient Care

- Determine the name of the hazardous material. If unable to determine material, contact the Chemical Transportation Emergency Center (CHEMTREC) at 1-800-262-8200, or reference the *Emergency Response Guidebook (ERG)*.
- Advise medical command of the material involved and request direction for treatment.

- The HAZMAT team and fire department are responsible for initial decontamination and patient packaging.
- Don personal protective equipment, as directed.
- Receive packaged patient at decontamination corridor from HAZMAT team and fire department and transfer to a prepared ambulance.
- Treat patient as directed by HAZMAT team and fire department.

Ambulance Preparation

- Prepare ambulance, as directed by HAZMAT team.
- Remove all nonessential supplies/equipment.
- Drape interior and floor with plastic, if directed.

Transport

- Notify receiving facility. Provide relevant information and ask where they would like you to park.
- After transferring the patient to emergency department (ED) staff, return to the ambulance. Do not move vehicle or allow others inside.
- Contact Incident Command to determine how and where the vehicle should be decontaminated.

EMS Personnel Exposure

- If exposed at the scene, remove yourself from further contamination and report the incident to the Safety Officer or HAZMAT team and wait for direction.
- After decontamination, receive clearance from HAZMAT team supervisor or ED MD and your supervisor before returning to duty.

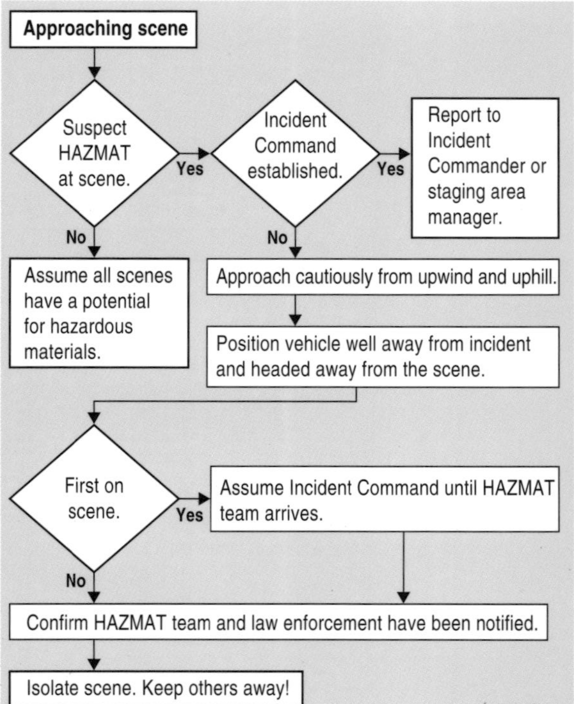
Approaching scene
Suspect HAZMAT at scene.
Yes
No
Assume all scenes have a potential for hazardous materials.
Incident Command established.
Yes
Report to Incident Commander or staging area manager.
No
Approach cautiously from upwind and uphill.
Position vehicle well away from incident and headed away from the scene.
First on scene.
Yes
Assume Incident Command until HAZMAT team arrives.
No
Confirm HAZMAT team and law enforcement have been notified.
Isolate scene. Keep others away!

continues

Patient care

↓

Determine material involved from HAZMAT team.

↓

Advise medical command of material involved and request direction for treatment.

↓

HAZMAT or fire personnel are responsible for initial decontamination and patient packaging.

↓

Don personal protective equipment as directed by HAZMAT team.

↓

Receive packaged patient at decontamination corridor from HAZMAT or fire department and transfer to prepared ambulance.

↓

Treat as directed by HAZMAT team, fire department, and medical command.

Ambulance preparation

↓

Prepare ambulance as directed by HAZMAT team.

↓

Remove all nonessential supplies/equipment.

Drape interior and floor of vehicle with plastic as directed.

Transport

Notify receiving facility: Provide relevant information and ask where they would like you to park.

Do not enter the ED without specific direction from the ED staff.

After transferring the patient to ED staff, return to the ambulance and remain inside. Do not move the vehicle or allow others inside.

Contact Incident Commander to determine how and where the vehicle should be decontaminated.

EMS personnel exposure

If exposed at scene: Remove yourself from further contamination and report incident to Safety Officer or HAZMAT team and wait for direction.

If exposed en route to the hospital: Inform ED and await direction.

continues

↓

After decontamination and treatment, receive clearance from HAZMAT team supervisor or ED MD and your supervisor before returning to duty.

Documentation

- Patient care
- Hazardous material present
- Communication with HAZMAT team and ED
- Measures taken to limit exposure
- Decontamination

Mass Casualty Incident

Mass Casualty Incidents

A mass casualty incident (MCI) is an event in which the number of patients exceeds the available resources in the initial response. By using the Incident Command System (ICS) and understanding the various roles and responsibilities of each person, the responders and/or the Incident Commander (IC) can manage the incident in a smooth, organized manner. All systems have different protocols for when to declare an MCI and initiate the ICS.

Medical Incident Command

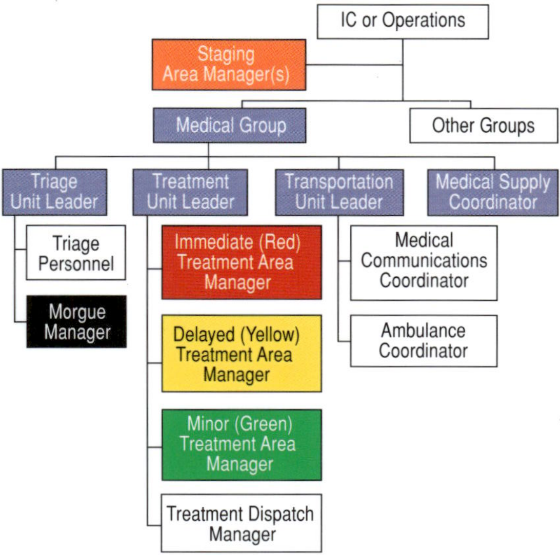

Triage Unit Leader

- Ensures safety of members working in the area.
- Counts and prioritizes patients using triage tags.
- Ensures all patients are moved to the treatment area.
- Documents activities in the triage area.
- Establishes initial morgue, if necessary.

Treatment Unit Leader

- Ensures safety of members working in the area.
- Sets up the treatment area with a tier for each triage level.
- Assign crews to treat patients.
- Ensures sufficient supplies and personnel.
- Initiates decontamination procedures, if necessary.
- Documents activities in the treatment area.

Transportation Unit Leader

- Ensures safety of members working in the area.
- Coordinates the transportation and destination of patients.
- Communicates with hospitals.
- Establishes a landing zone for air medical, if needed.
- Tracks all patient movement.

Triage

Triage simply means to "sort" your patients based on the severity of their injuries.

Triage Categories

There are five common triage categories:

Immediate (red tag): First-priority patients need immediate care and transport. They usually have problems with ABCs, head trauma, or shock. Patients who fall into this category have respirations > 30 breaths/min; capillary refill > 2 seconds; no radial pulse; and are unable are to follow simple commands.

Delayed (yellow tag): Second-priority patients who need care and transport but can be delayed.

Minor (green tag): Third-priority patients are ambulatory and need minimal treatment.

Deceased (black tag): No respirations after the head tilt–chin lift procedure is performed.

Uninjured (white tag): These victims do not need or want medical assistance. They are not entered into the EMS system but still need to be documented.

NJ Triage Tags

When a triage system is used, it is vital that there is some way for responders to keep an accurate record of patients' conditions. Triage tags are used to clearly show the category of each patient. Triage tags are usually used when there are eight (8) or more minor (green) patients, when there are six (6) or more patients with mixed categories, or when there are four (4) or more immediate (red) patients. Each unit is required to carry a minimum of 50 triage tags at all times. Triage tags are double-sided.

Personal Property/ Evidence Tag — *Attach stub or seal inside personal property or evidence bag*

Patient Destination and Transport Unit — *Remove this stub after arrival at hospital and keep until attached to patient care report*

PEEL AND STICK TO ◯ PATIENT CHART

RESPIRATIONS	PERFUSION	MENTAL STATUS
R ☐ Yes ☐ No	P ☐ Pulse ☐ No	M ☐ Can Do ☐ Can't Do

Move ANYONE ambulatory	⇨ MINOR
No Respiration after head tilt	⇨ DECEASED
Respirations OVER 30	⇨ IMMEDIATE
No radial pulse or Capillary refill over 2 Seconds	⇨ IMMEDIATE
Unable to follow simple commands	⇨ IMMEDIATE
Everyone else	⇨ DELAYED

☐ S Salivation ☐ L Lacrimation ☐ U Urination ☐ D Defecation ☐ G GI Distress ☐ E Emesis ☐ M Miosis

NAAK AUTO INJECTOR ☐ 1 ☐ 2 ☐ 3 ☐ 4 ☐ 5

☐ Dry Decon
☐ Gross Decon
☐ Technical Decon
Decon Solution____________

Circle Nature of Contaminant

Vitals

Time	B/P	Pulse	Resp	O_2 Sat

Medications

Time	Medication	Dose	Route

IV Location______ Ga.______ Solution:______ Rate:______

Airway Adjunct______ Size:______ Depth.______

STATE OF NEW JERSEY

DECEASED

IMMEDIATE
LIFE THREATENING INJURIES

DELAYED
NON-LIFE THREATENING INJURIES

MINOR
MINOR INJURIES

UNINJURED
DOCUMENTED BY OFFICIAL

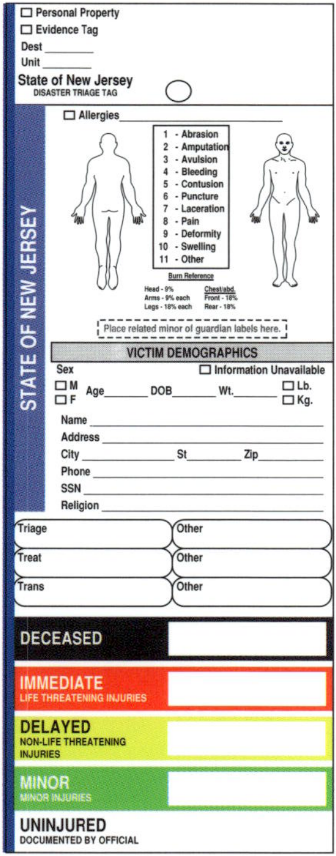

☐ Personal Property
☐ Evidence Tag
Dest ________
Unit ________

State of New Jersey
DISASTER TRIAGE TAG

STATE OF NEW JERSEY

☐ Allergies ____________________

1 - Abrasion
2 - Amputation
3 - Avulsion
4 - Bleeding
5 - Contusion
6 - Puncture
7 - Laceration
8 - Pain
9 - Deformity
10 - Swelling
11 - Other

Burn Reference
Head - 9%
Arms - 9% each
Legs - 18% each
Chest/abd.
Front - 18%
Rear - 18%

Place related minor of guardian labels here.

VICTIM DEMOGRAPHICS

Sex ☐ Information Unavailable
☐ M ☐ F Age______ DOB______ Wt.______ ☐ Lb. ☐ Kg.
Name ____________________
Address ____________________
City ____________ St ________ Zip ________
Phone ____________________
SSN ____________________
Religion ____________________

Triage	Other
Treat	Other
Trans	Other

DECEASED

IMMEDIATE
LIFE THREATENING INJURIES

DELAYED
NON-LIFE THREATENING INJURIES

MINOR
MINOR INJURIES

UNINJURED
DOCUMENTED BY OFFICIAL

Determining a Patient's Priority

START Triage

START triage is one of the easiest methods of triage. START stands for Simple Triage And Rapid Treatment. This method gives you the ability to rapidly categorize patients at an MCI. The staff members at Hoag Memorial Hospital, Newport Beach, California, are responsible for developing this method.

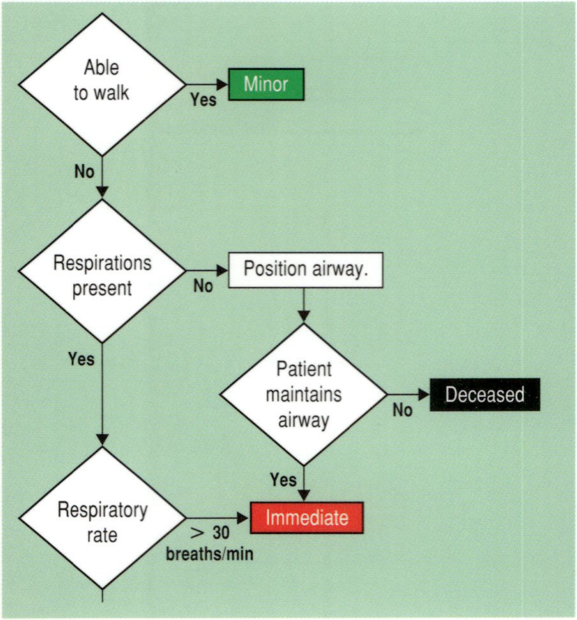

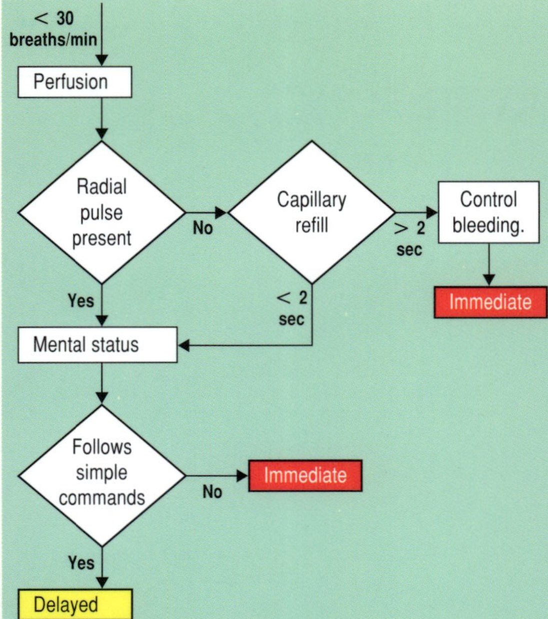

The clinician should view this protocol as an adjunct to your system's disaster plan only if START triage is a part of that plan. This protocol does not constitute or attempt to substitute for a disaster plan and should be used only in conjunction with the system-wide response approved in your area.

JumpSTART Triage

The JumpSTART triage method was developed by Lou Romig, MD. This method takes into account the physiologic and developmental differences of pediatric patients. This method is intended to be used for patients younger than 8 years who appear to weigh less than 100 lb.

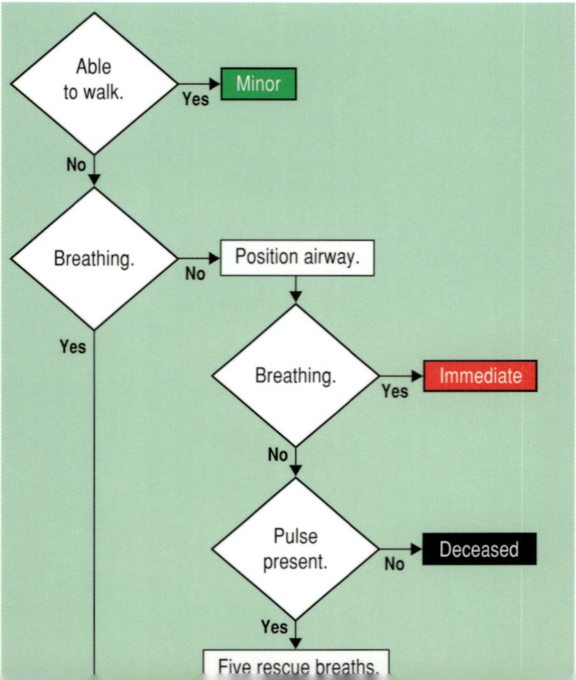

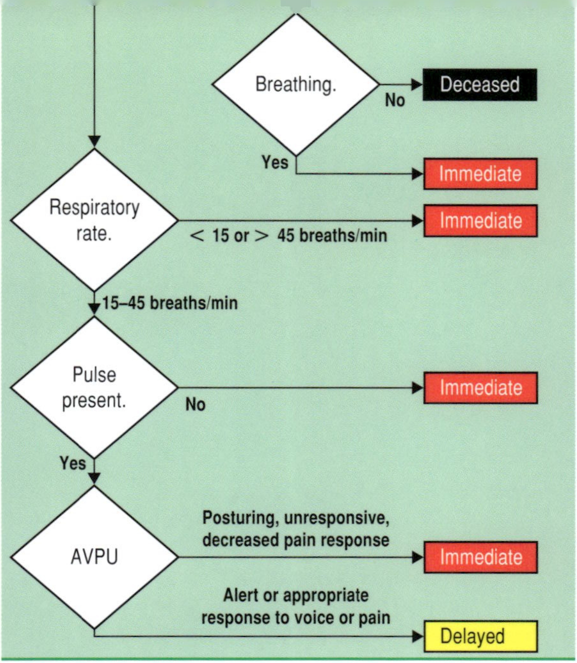

Changing a Patient's Priority

To change a patient's condition:

1. Leave the original triage tag on the patient.
2. Retag the patient with a new triage tag.
3. Write a large "2" on the new triage tag.
4. Additional, successive retriaging should be numbered sequentially (3, 4, 5).

NJ Burn Matrix for Mass Casualties

Once a burn mass casualty incident has been declared, triage burn patients following the NJ Burn Matrix for Mass Casualties:

Tier I (red)	Survival and good outcome likely (survival > 50%) with aggressive care and comprehensive resources)
Tier II (yellow)	Survival and good outcome likely (survival > 90% with limited/short term admission and resources)
Tier II/Tier III (blue)	Survival and good outcome likely (survival < 50%) even with long-term, aggressive treatment and resources)
Outpatient (green)	Survival and good outcome expected without requiring initial admission
Tier IV (gray)	Survival less than 10% even with unlimited, aggressive treatment

New Jersey Burn Tier Matrix of Patient Distribution for Mass Casualties

Burn with Smoke Inhalation		0-10%	11-20%	21-30%	31-40%	41-50%	51-60%	61-70%	71 80%	> 80%
% TBSA / AGE	0-10%	11-20%	21-30 %	31-40 %	41-50 %	51-60%	61-70%	71-80%	81-90%	90+%
0-1 Y	Tier II	Tier II	Tier I	Tier I	Tier I	Tier I	Tier III Tier II	Tier III Tier II	Tier III Tier II	Tier IV
2-4 Y	Outpatient	Tier II	Tier II	Tier I	Tier I	Tier I	Tier I	Tier III Tier II	Tier III Tier II	Tier III Tier II
5-19 Y	Outpatient	Tier II	Tier II	Tier II	Tier I	Tier I	Tier I	Tier I	Tier I	Tier III Tier II
20-29 Y	Outpatient	Tier II	Tier II	Tier II	Tier I	Tier I	Tier I	Tier I	Tier III Tier II	Tier III Tier II
30-39 Y	Outpatient	Tier II	Tier II	Tier I	Tier I	Tier I	Tier I	Tier I	Tier III Tier II	Tier III Tier II
40-49 Y	Outpatient	Tier II	Tier II	Tier I	Tier I	Tier I	Tier I	Tier III Tier II	Tier III Tier II	Tier III Tier II
50-59 Y	Outpatient	Tier II	Tier II	Tier I	Tier I	Tier I	Tier III Tier II	Tier III Tier II	Tier IV	Tier IV
60-69 Y	Tier II	Tier II	Tier I	Tier I	Tier I	Tier III Tier II	Tier III Tier II	Tier III Tier II	Tier IV	Tier IV
70+ Y	Tier II	Tier I	Tier I	Tier III Tier II	Tier III Tier II	Tier IV	Tier IV	Tier IV	Tier IV	Tier IV

Tier I: Burn Centers Tier II: NJ Trauma Centers Tier III: Medical Centers >250 beds Tier IV: Community Hospital <250 beds

Patient Survivability: GREEN – Stable YELLOW – High RED – Medium PURPLE – Low GRAY - Expectar

Personal Protective Equipment

Personal protective equipment (PPE) is clothing and gear designed to create a barrier against workplace hazards, as well as to prevent injury from incorrect use or malfunction of equipment. Examples include gloves, gowns, respirators, face shields, and reflective vests.

Using Personal Protective Equipment

TABLE 1 Tasks Requiring Personal Protective Equipment

Component	Task
Hand hygiene 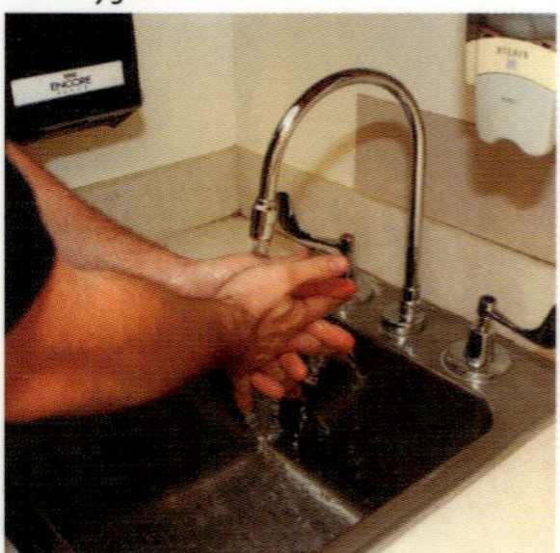	Wash hands: • For at least 30 seconds. • After touching blood, body fluids, secretions, excretions, or contaminated items. • Immediately after removing gloves. • Between patient contacts.

Personal Protective Equipment (PPE)

Gloves

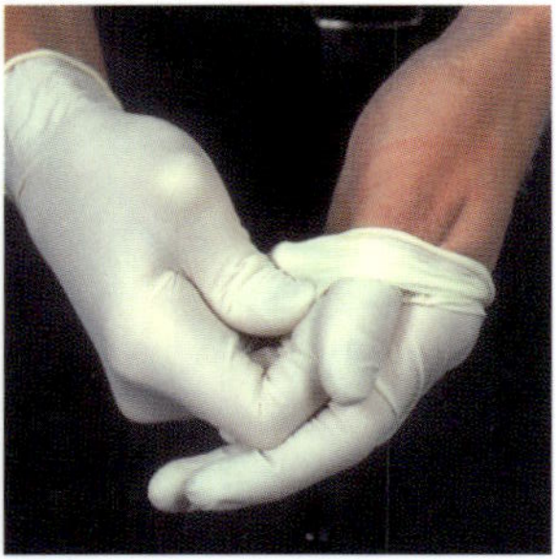

- For touching blood, body fluids, secretions, excretions, or contaminated items.
- For touching mucous membranes and non-intact skin.
- Remove gloves when not providing patient care.

Gown

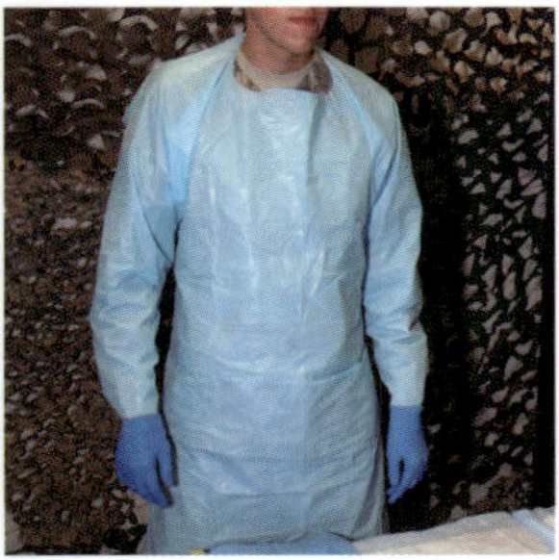

- During procedures and patient care activities when contact of the responder's clothing/exposed skin to blood, body fluids, secretions, excretions, or contaminated items is anticipated.

continues

TABLE 1 Tasks Requiring Personal Protective Equipment, continued

Component	Task
Mask, face shield combination 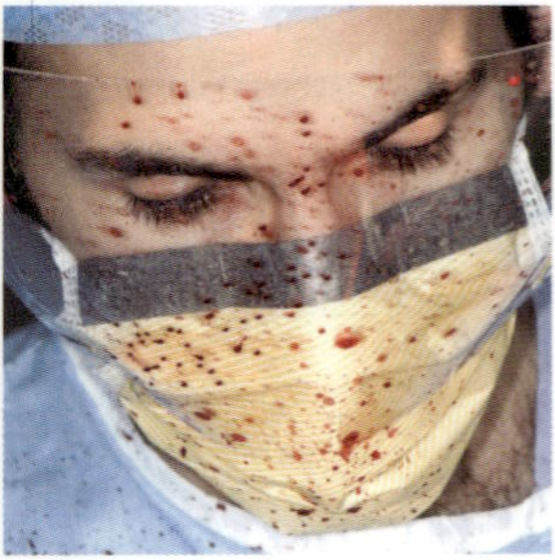	• During procedures and patient care activities likely to generate splashes or sprays of blood, body fluids, secretions, or excretions. Examples include suctioning or endotracheal intubation.
Facemask 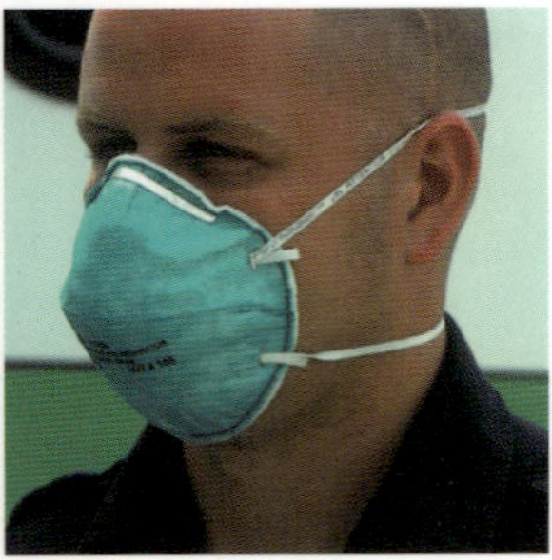	• Helps to block large-particle droplets, splashes, sprays, or splatter that may contain germs.

N-95 Particulate Respirator

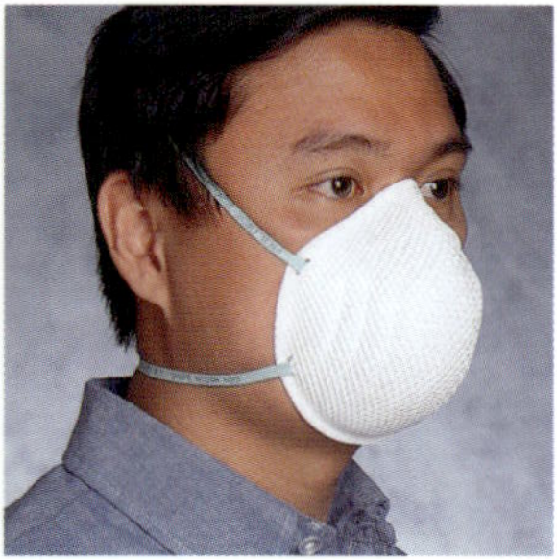

- Respiratory protective device.
- Designed to prevent inhalation of very small particles.
- Blocks at least 95% of airborne particles.

Patient Care Environment

Environmental controls

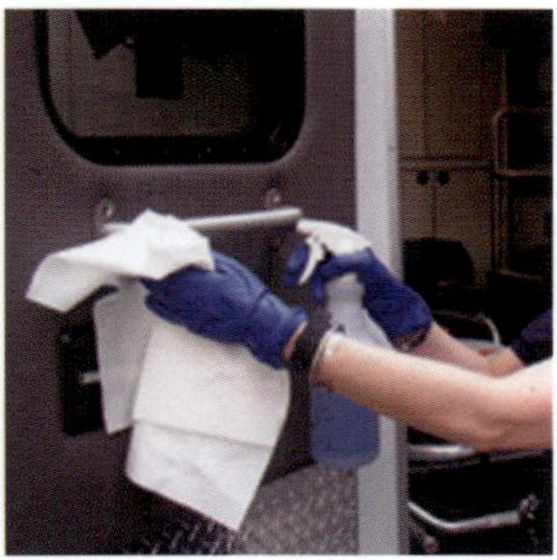

- Have procedures for the routine care, cleaning, and disinfection of environmental surfaces.
- Pay special attention to frequently touched surfaces within the ambulance (handrails, seats, cabinets, doors).

continues

TABLE 1 Tasks Requiring Personal Protective Equipment, continued

Component	Task
Textiles and laundry 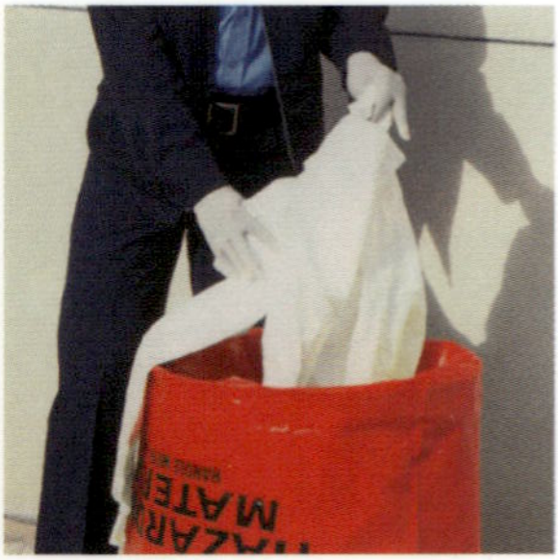	• Handle in a manner that prevents transfer of microorganisms to others and to the environment.
Needles and other sharp objects 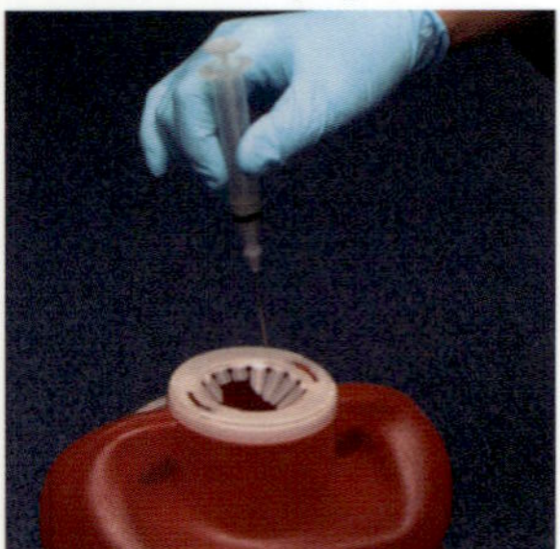	• Do not recap, bend, break, or hand manipulate used needles. • Use safety features when available (needleless vascular access systems). • Place sharps in puncture-resistant containers.

Special Circumstances

Patient resuscitation

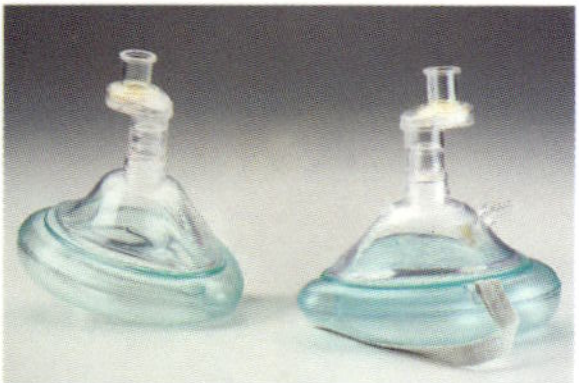

- Use mouthpiece, resuscitation bag, or other ventilation devices to prevent contact with mouth and oral secretions.

Respiratory hygiene/cough etiquette

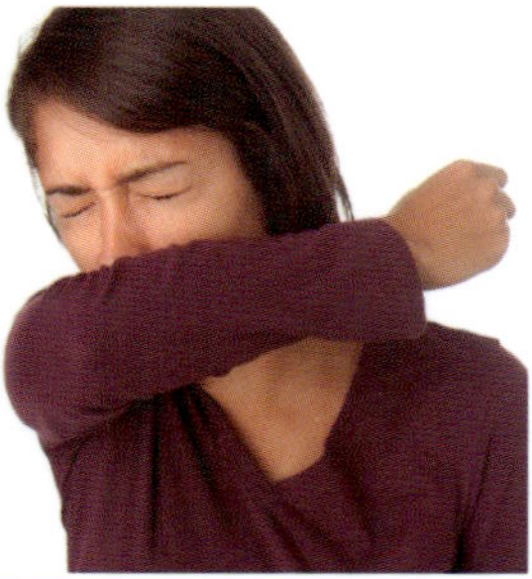

- Instruct symptomatic patients to cover mouth/nose when sneezing or coughing.
- Use tissues and dispose in no-touch receptacle.
- Perform hand hygiene after touching tissues.
- Place surgical mask on patient/provider.
- If mask cannot be used, maintain spacial separation (> 3 feet), if possible.

How to Properly Don and Doff PPE

Don and doff PPE in the order shown in **Table 2.***

TABLE 2 Donning and Doffing PPE

Don Process	Doff Process
1. Gown • Select appropriate type and size. • Opening should be in the back. • Secure at neck and waist. • If gown is too small, use two (tie one in front and one in back).	**1. Gloves** • Grasp outside edge near wrist. • Peel away from hand, turning glove inside out. • Hold in opposite gloved hand. • Slide ungloved finger under the wrist of remaining glove. • Peel off from inside, creating a bag for both gloves and discard.
2. Mask or particulate respirator Mask • Place mask over nose, mouth, chin. • Fit flexible nose piece over nose bridge. • Secure on head with ties or elastic. • Adjust to fit. Particulate respirator (must be fit-tested annually) • Select fit-tested respirator. • Hold N-95 in hand (narrow end at fingertips). • Place N-95 under chin.	**2. Goggles or face shield** • Grasp ear or head pieces with ungloved hands. • Lift away from face. • Place on designated receptacle for reprocessing or disposal.

Don Process	Doff Process
2. Particulate respirator, continued • Place top strap on top of head, bottom strap below ear. • Adjust to fit. • Perform a fit check (inhaling should collapse the mask, exhale to check for leaks).	
3. Goggles or face shield • Position goggles over eyes and secure to the head using the ear pieces of headband. • Position face shield over face and secure on brow with headband. • Adjust to fit comfortably.	**3. Gown** • Unfasten ties. • Peel gown away from neck and shoulder. • Turn the contaminated outside of gown toward the inside. • Fold or roll into a bundle. • Discard in red biohazard bag.
4. Gloves • Don gloves last. • Select correct type and size. • Insert hands into gloves. • Extend gloves over isolation gown cuffs.	**4. Mask or particulate respirator** Mask • Untie the bottom, then the top. • Remove from face. • Discard. Particulate respirator • Remove the bottom strap first, then the top. • Remove from face. • Discard. • Thoroughly wash hands with soap and water.

* Combination of PPE will affect sequence. Be practical!

PPE Tips

- **Be safe**. If you think a patient might have an infectious condition or be contaminated, treat the patient as such until proven otherwise. Request appropriate PPE and resources if they are not available at the scene.
- **Vaccinate**. Be up-to-date on all vaccinations, including hepatitis B and influenza.
- **Wash your hands**. Wash your hands throughout the day and after every patient contact. Use an alcohol-based hand sanitizer if you don't have access to soap and water.

Adapted from: Department of Health and Senior Services, Office of Emergency Medical Services, and Public Employees Occupational Safety and Health (PEOSH) Administration, *Personal Protective Equipment for EMS Agencies*, flyer.

Terrorism and Weapons of Mass Destruction

Terrorism

Terrorism is the use of violence against persons or property in violation of the criminal laws of the United States for purposes of intimidation, coercion, or ransom. Terrorism aims to:

- Create fear among the public.
- Convince citizens that their government is powerless to prevent terrorism.
- Get immediate publicity for their causes.

Terrorism may be accomplished through kidnappings, assassinations, hijackings, bomb scares and bombings, cyber attacks, and the use of chemical, biologic, radiologic, nuclear, and explosive weapons.

The number of the toll -free, 24-hour Terrorism Hotline is **1-866-4SAFENJ**.

Weapons of Mass Destruction

A weapon of mass destruction (WMD) is any agent designed to bring about mass death, casualties, and/or massive damage to property and infrastructure (bridges, tunnels, airports, and seaports). These instruments of death and destruction include biologic, nuclear, incendiary, chemical, and explosive weapons (B-NICE) or chemical, biologic, radiologic, nuclear, and explosive (CBRNE) weapons. Both mnemonics (B-NICE and CBRNE) are used to remember the kinds of weapons of mass destruction.

Chemical Agents

TABLE 1 Types of Chemical Agents

Chemical Agent	Signs and Symptoms	Treatment
Nerve agents: Tabun (GA) Sarin (GB) Soman (GD) VX	Rhinorrhea, dyspnea, apnea, convulsions, paralysis, altered mental status, excessive secretions. Odor: fruity (GA, GB, GD), sulfur (VX)	Decontaminate and call for ALS and HAZMAT. No decontamination needed for exposure to vapor. Secure ABCs.*
Vesicants (blister agents): Sulfur mustard (H) Lewisite (L) Phosgene oxime (CX)	Asymptomatic latent period, skin redness (erythema) and blisters, upper respiratory secretions, dyspnea, airway damage, gastrointestinal effects. Odor: garlic (H), geraniums (L)	There are no antidotes. British anti-Lewisite is the antidote for Lewisite; however, it is not carried by civilian EMS. Decontaminate before initiating ABCs. Patient may require prompt airway support if agent is inhaled. Transport as soon as possible.
Metabolic agents: Hydrogen cyanide (AC) Cyanogen chloride (CK)	After exposure to high estimated dose: seizures, cardiopulmonary arrest. Odor: bitter almonds (AC), irritating (CK)	Ensure decontamination has been performed. Remove patient from atmosphere. Support ABCs. Mild-exposure (conscious) patients: do not receive an antidote; provide 100% oxygen and suction, as needed. Severe-exposure (unconscious and/or not breathing) patients: secure airway, provide oxygen and

Chemical Agent	Signs and Symptoms	Treatment
Metabolic agents, continued:		perhaps ventilation with supplemental oxygen via bag-valve-mask device or ventilator device. Also, see *Cyanide Exposure and Treatment* protocol.
Pulmonary agents (choking agents): Phosgene (CG) Chlorine (CL)	Immediate burning and irritation followed by wheal-like lesions, eye and airway damage. Odor: freshly mown hay or grass (CG), bleach (CL)	Remove patient from contaminated atmosphere; decontaminate; treat ABCs aggressively; suction as necessary; place patient in position of comfort with head elevated; initiate rapid transport. There are no antidotes to counteract these agents.
Neurotoxin agents: Ricin	Initial symptoms will develop 6–8 hours after exposure: respiratory distress, fever, cough, nausea, chest tightness, vomiting, diarrhea, erythema, and severe diaphoresis.	Treatment is supportive and includes respiratory support and cardiovascular support, as needed. Early intubation and ventilation, combined with treatment of pulmonary edema, are appropriate. There is no treatment or vaccine available.

*Note: The DuoDote Auto-Injector contains 2.1 mg of atropine and 600 mg of 2-PAM delivered in a single dose through one needle.

First responders must be familiar with the SLUDGEM mnemonic to accurately identify the signs and symptoms of a nerve agent or organophosphate exposure:

S—Salivation
L—Lacrimation
U—Urination
D—Defecation
G—Gastric emptying
E—Emesis
M—Miosis

Biologic Agents

Table 2 shows only a handful of the biologic agents prehospital care providers may encounter in the field. The prehospital treatment of these agents is mostly supportive.

TABLE 2 Biologic Agents

Biologic Agents	Signs and Symptoms	Treatment
Anthrax Cholera Q fever Tularemia	Fever, general malaise and weakness, flulike symptoms, chest discomfort, cough, dyspnea, diaphoresis, signs of shock, organ and system failure, death	*Pulmonary/inhalation*: Follow standard precautions, oxygen, ventilatory support if in pulmonary edema or respiratory failure, and transport. *Cutaneous:* Follow standard precautions; apply dry, sterile dressing to prevent accidental contact with wound and fluids.

Biologic Agents	Signs and Symptoms	Treatment
Botulinum toxin	Dry mouth, intestinal obstruction, urinary retention, constipation, nausea, vomiting, abnormal pupil dilation, blurred and/or double vision, drooping eyelids, difficulty swallowing and/or speaking, respiratory failure as result of descending paralysis.	Support ABCs, provide oxygen, transport, ventilatory support in case of paralysis of the respiratory muscles. Botulism anti-toxin is available.
Smallpox	Severe fever, malaise, body aches, headaches, small blisters on skin, bleeding of skin and mucous membranes.	Follow standard precautions, support ABCs. There is no specific treatment.
Tuberculosis Plague	Above symptoms with hemoptysis, lymph tenderness.	Follow standard precautions, support ABCs, provide oxygen, transport.

Personal protective equipment is to be used when treating any patient suspected of being exposed to a biologic agent.

Radiologic/Nuclear

Table 3 describes the radiologic and nuclear incidents that prehospital care providers may see in the field and their appropriate treatments.

- Radiologic: Energy in the form of waves or particles. Radiation comes from sources such as radioactive material or from equipment such as x-ray machines.
- Nuclear: A weapon whose destructive power derives from an uncontrolled nuclear reactive.

All nuclear explosions result in the dispersal of radiologic agents. However, not all radiation originates from a nuclear explosion.

TABLE 3 Radiologic Incidents

Radiologic Agents	
Symptoms of high level of exposure	Nonspecific; usually include anorexia, nausea, vomiting, skin erythema (redness). Patients may exhibit intermittent periods of overall well-being. However, this can be short-lived, and patients will begin exhibiting worsening signs and symptoms. Patients can succumb after a few hours, but could live up to several months.
Treatment	Exposure to radiation source does not make a patient contaminated or radioactive. When radioactive source is physically on the body, the patient is contaminated and must be decontaminated. Once decontaminated, direct attention to physical injuries from the blast and management of ABCs. Transport.
Factors affecting exposure	Exposures are related to distance, time, and shielding. Patients exposed to radiation in either large doses or for an extended period of time will exhibit more severe signs and symptoms.

Incendiary and Explosive Devices

The type and severity of wounds sustained from incendiary and explosive devices primarily depend on the patient's distance from the epicenter of the explosion.

TABLE 4 The Anatomy of an Explosion

Phase	Injuries
Primary blast injury	Direct effects of the pressure wave on body. Mostly affects gas-filled organs such as lungs, intestines, and middle ear.
Secondary blast injury	Penetrating or nonpenetrating injury that results from being struck by flying debris. May cause both penetrating and/or blunt trauma.
Tertiary blast injury	Whole body displacement or body being thrown and subsequent traumatic impact with environmental objects. This results in a wide array of injuries, including blunt trauma and even penetrating trauma, such as impalement.
Quaternary blast injuries	Associated injuries not due to primary, secondary, or tertiary mechanisms. Thermal and inhalation injuries as well as crush injuries.

Secondary Devices

First responders must be vigilant when responding to a reported explosion due to the possible presence of "secondary devices." These devices are bombs placed at the scene before the first explosion, but detonated afterward with the intention of killing first responders. In addition, an improvised explosive device (IED) can be combined with any of the other weapons of mass destruction to create a "dirty bomb." In the case of radiologic and biologic agents, first responders may not know they have been exposed until after the incident has ended.

Vehicle-Borne Improvised Explosive Device (IED) Identification

The following may indicate a vehicle carrying an IED:

- A vehicle that is heavy or sagging (rear-weighted).
- A vehicle that is parked illegally or near authorized vehicle entrances or crowded access points.
- A vehicle with covered or tinted windows.
- A vehicle with large containers on seats or cargo area (e.g., bags, boxes, barrels, tanks).
- A vehicle without a license plate or that has a plate that has been altered.
- Odor of gasoline, propane, acids, or chemicals.
- Visible wires, switches, batteries, or antennae inside or on a vehicle.
- Cargo concealed with tarp or blanket.

If observed, call dispatch or communications center.

Cyanide Exposure and Treatment

Considerations

The following standing orders (optional, at medical director's discretion) are authorized in the event an adult patient presents with cyanide poisoning.

Assessment

- There may be no distinguishing physical findings or symptoms, particularly at low concentrations.
- There may be rapid death in high concentrations. Sudden collapse, seizures, or death after exposure. Generally, the victims are acyanotic (often retain the normal pink coloration until after death).
- There may be an odor of bitter almonds. Victims often will complain of dizziness, weakness, and anxiety.
- Determine level of exposure:
  - *If the exposure level is mild (patient is conscious and breathing):* Secure airway. Give oxygen 100%. Observe for respiratory distress. Suction, as needed.
  - *If the exposure level is severe (patient is unconscious or respirations are severely compromised):* Secure airway. Give oxygen 100%. Suction, as needed.
- BLS to request ALS and HAZMAT.

Treatment

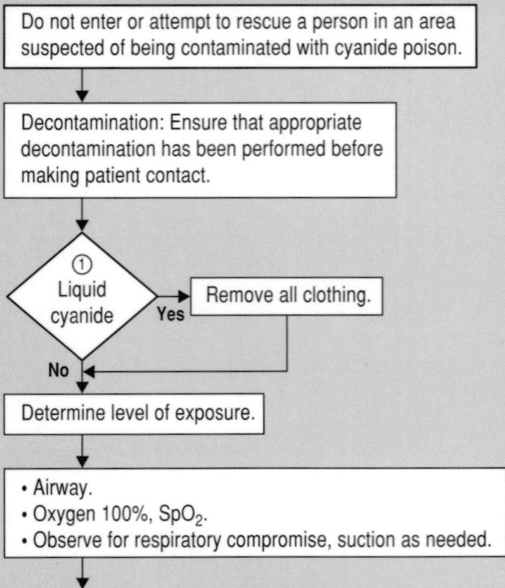
Do not enter or attempt to rescue a person in an area suspected of being contaminated with cyanide poison.
Decontamination: Ensure that appropriate decontamination has been performed before making patient contact.
① Liquid cyanide
Yes
Remove all clothing.
No
Determine level of exposure.
• Airway.
• Oxygen 100%, SpO_2.
• Observe for respiratory compromise, suction as needed.

(2) Severe exposure.

- **Yes** →

If using CYANOKIT ®:

1. Establish vascular access.
2. Add 100 mL NS injection to first CYANOKIT vial per transfer spike.
3. Mix CYANOKIT vial for 30 seconds. Do not shake.
4. Use vented IV tubing to infuse over 7.5 minutes.
5. Repeat steps 1–3 for second vial.
6. Contact medical command physician.

If using cyanide kit:

1. Break/hold an aspirol of amyl nitrate in front of the patient's nose for 15 seconds, remove for 15 seconds.
2. Use a new aspirol of amyl nitrate every 3 minutes thereafter, until vascular access is established. If unconscious, place the aspirol in the mask of the bag-valve-mask device.
3. Give sodium thiosulfate 12.5 g IV when vascular access established.
4. Contact medical command physician.

- **No** → Cardiac monitor. → Transport.

1. No decontamination is needed if exposure is pure vapor cyanide.
2. Severe exposure: The patient is unconscious or in respiratory compromise.

Documentation

- Signs and symptoms
- Cardiac rhythm, if obtained
- Nature of exposure
- Response to treatment

Organophosphate Exposure

Considerations

Organophosphate is a family of nerve agents. Examples include the following:

- **Insecticides**: malathion, parathion, diazinon, fenthion, dichlorvos, chlorpyrifos, ethion
- **Nerve gases**: soman, sarin, tabun, VX
- **Antihelmintics**: trichlorfon
- **Herbicides**: tribufos (DEF), merphos, tricresyl phosphate

Assessment

- Signs and symptoms include sudden collapse, seizures, muscle fasciculations (contractions), cyanosis, bradycardia, miosis (small pupils), shortness of breath, cough, excess nasal secretions, excess pulmonary secretions, salivation, urination, nausea, vomiting, diarrhea, headache, muscle weakness, blurred or dimmed vision.
- Effects appear almost immediately and will vary from mild to severe. There will likely be deaths near the source of the exposure.
- Do not enter or attempt to rescue a person in an area suspected of being contaminated with organophosphate.
- Decontamination: Before making patient contact, ensure that appropriate decontamination has been performed. If it is certain the exposure is to gas, there is no need for decontamination. If there is the possibility of droplet or liquid contamination, ensure that all clothing is removed.
- BLS to request ALS and HAZMAT.
- Airway, oxygen 100%.
- Suction, as needed.

Treatment

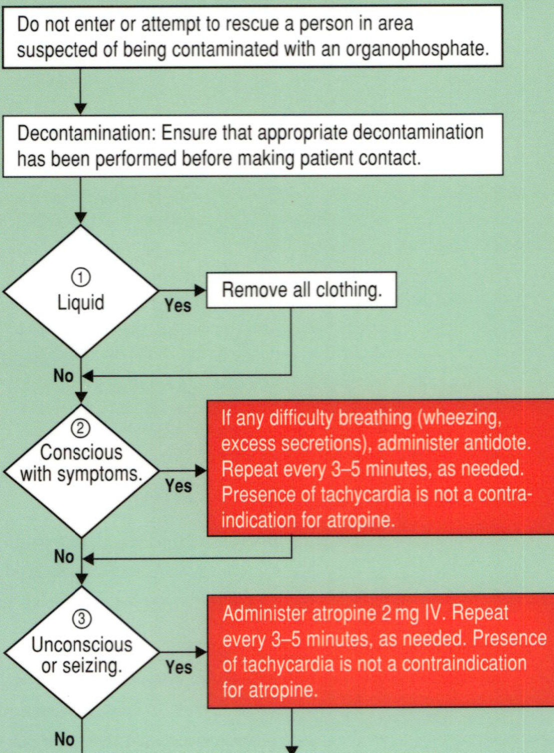
Do not enter or attempt to rescue a person in area suspected of being contaminated with an organophosphate.
Decontamination: Ensure that appropriate decontamination has been performed before making patient contact.
① Liquid
Yes
Remove all clothing.
No
② Conscious with symptoms.
Yes
If any difficulty breathing (wheezing, excess secretions), administer antidote. Repeat every 3–5 minutes, as needed. Presence of tachycardia is not a contra-indication for atropine.
No
③ Unconscious or seizing.
Yes
Administer atropine 2 mg IV. Repeat every 3–5 minutes, as needed. Presence of tachycardia is not a contraindication for atropine.
No

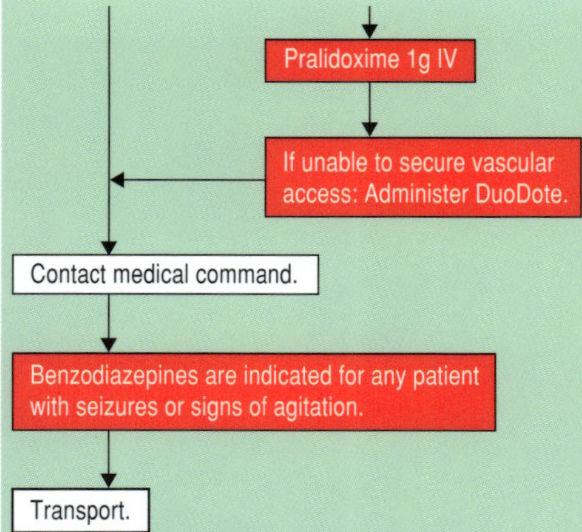

1. No decontamination is needed if exposure is a pure vapor.
2. Conscious and breathing, but symptomatic.
3. Unconscious, seizing, postictal, not breathing, or with symptoms of two or more organs.

Pediatric Considerations

ALS

Atropine: 0.02 mg/kg IV/IO with a minimum of 0.1 mg and maximum of 0.5 mg as the first dose. If patient is older than 10 years, treat as an adult. If IV/IO access is not available and the child is seriously ill, a single IM dose of atropine 2 mg is acceptable. Children younger than 2 years of age should be initially dosed at 0.1 mg and titrated to effect (dry secretions).

Pralidoxime: Smaller children should be treated intravenously, if possible, at a dose of 25–50 mg/kg up to 1–2 grams given as a 5% solution or less over no faster than 20–30 minutes. If vascular access is not available, a single dose of 600 mg IM is acceptable in any child above 10 kg. Even smaller children may be treated based on urgency.

Documentation

- Signs and symptoms
- Cardiac rhythm, if obtained
- Nature of exposure
- Treatment
- Response to treatment

Anatomy References

Planes of the Body

The anatomic planes of the body are imaginary straight lines that divide the body. There are three main axes of the body, depending on how it is sliced.

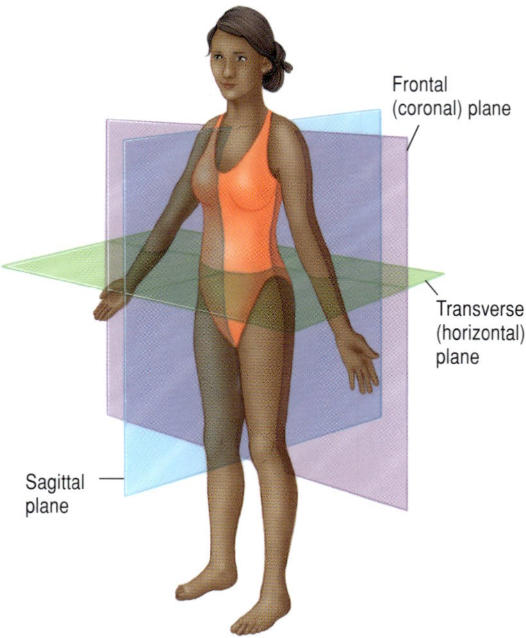

TABLE 1 Planes of the Body

Plane	Description
Coronal	Front and back
Transverse	Top and bottom
Sagittal	Left and right
Midsagittal (midline)	Left and right, equal halves

Directional Terms

When you are discussing where an injury is located or how a pain radiates in the body, you need to know the correct directional terms.

Table 2 provides the basic directional terms used in medicine. Directional terms are paired as "opposites."

TABLE 2 Common Directional Terms

Common Term	Directional Term	Definition
Front and back	Anterior (ventral)	The front surface of the body
	Posterior (dorsal)	The back surface of the patient
Right and left	Right	The patient's right
	Left	The patient's left
Top and bottom	Superior	Closest to the head
	Inferior	Closest to the feet
Closest and farthest	Proximal	Closest to the point of attachment
	Distal	Farthest from the point of attachment
Middle and side	Medial	Closest to the midline
	Lateral	Farthest from the midline
In and out	Superficial	Closest to the surface of the skin
	Deep	Farthest from the surface of the skin

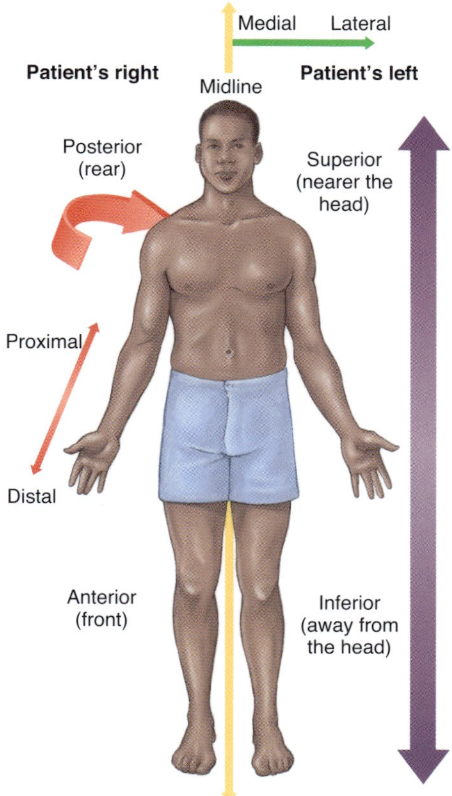
Medial
Lateral
Patient's right
Patient's left
Midline
Posterior
(rear)
Superior
(nearer the
head)
Proximal
Distal
Anterior
(front)
Inferior
(away from
the head)

Abdominal Quadrants

The sections of the abdominal cavity are described by quadrants.

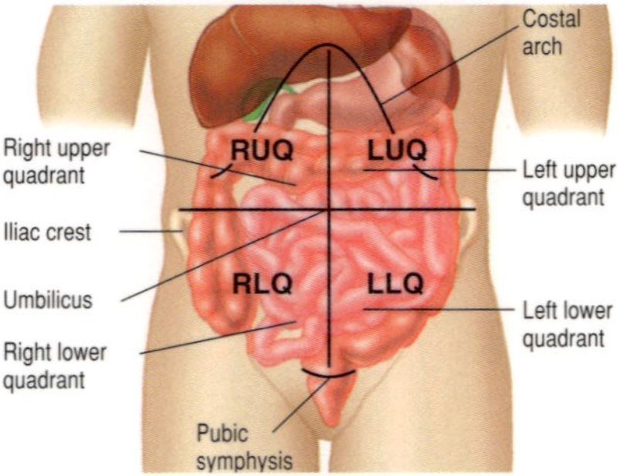

Right Upper Quadrant	Left Upper Quadrant
Liver	Left lower part of liver
Gallbladder	Upper lobe of left kidney
Duodenum	Splenic flexure of colon
Head of pancreas	Section of transverse colon
Right Adrenal gland	Section of descending colon
Upper lobe of right kidney	Stomach
Hepatic flexure of colon	Spleen
Section of ascending colon	Pancreas
Section of transverse colon	Left Adrenal gland
Right Lower Quadrant	**Left Lower Quadrant**
Lower lobe of right kidney	Lower lobe of left kidney
Section of ascending colon	Section of descending colon
Right fallopian tube (female)	Left spermatic cord (male)
Right ovary (female)	Part of uterus (if enlarged)
Part of uterus (if enlarged)	Sigmoid colon
Right spermatic cord (male)	Left ureter
Cecum	Left ovary (female)
Appendix	Left fallopian tube (female)
Right ureter	

Dermatome Chart

Dermatome: Distinct areas of skin that correspond to specific spinal or cranial nerve levels where sensory nerves enter the central nervous system.

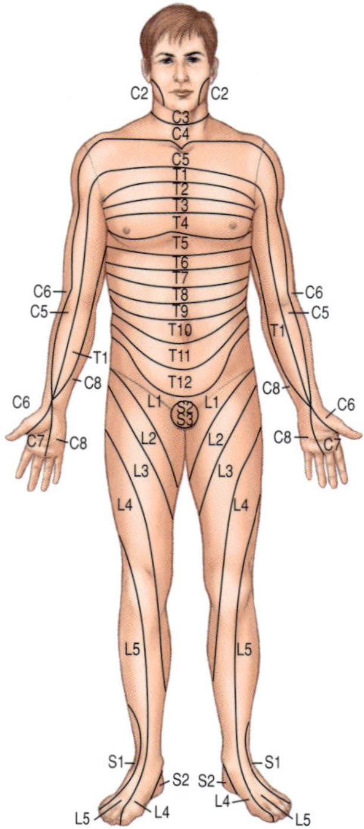

Common Medical Abbreviations

ABCs	airway, breathing, circulation
abd	abdomen
ACLS	advanced cardiac life support
ACS	acute coronary syndrome
AIDS	acquired immune deficiency syndrome
AMU	air medical unit
A & O	alert and oriented
ASA	aspirin
bid	twice a day
BM	bowel movement
BP	blood pressure
BSA	body surface area
BVM	bag-valve-mask
$\bar{c}$	with
CA	cancer
CABG	coronary artery bypass graft
CAD	coronary artery disease
CAP	capsule
CBC	complete blood count
CC	chief complaint
CHF	congestive heart failure
CID	cervical immobilization device
cm	centimeter
CNS	central nervous system
CO	carbon monoxide
CO_2	carbon dioxide
COPD	chronic obstructive pulmonary disease
CSF	cerebrospinal fluid
CVA	cerebrovascular accident (stroke)

D/C	discontinue
DKA	diabetic ketoacidosis
DNR	do not resuscitate
DOB	date of birth
Dx	diagnosis
ED	emergency department
ETT	endotracheal tube
ETA	estimated time of arrival
ETOH	alcohol
GCS	Glasgow Coma Scale
GI	gastrointestinal
GSW	gunshot wound
gt	drop
gtt	drops
GU	genitourinary
HIV	human immunodeficiency virus
HR	heart rate
hr (h)	hour
HTN	hypertension (high blood pressure)
Hx	history
IM	intramuscular
inj	injection; injury
IO	intraosseous
IV	intravenous
JVD	jugular vein distention
K^+	potassium
kg	kilogram
Ⓛ	left
L	liter
LBB	long backboard
LLQ	left lower quadrant

continues

LMP	last menstrual period
LOC	level of consciousness; loss of consciousness
lpm (LPM, L/min)	liters per minute
LR	lactated Ringer's
LUQ	left upper quadrant
m	meter
mcg	microgram
MCI	multiple casualty incident
mEq	milliequivalent
mg	milligram
MI	myocardial infarction (heart attack)
MICU	Mobile Intensive Care Unit
min	minute; minimum
mL	milliliter
mm	millimeter
MOI	mechanism of injury
Na	sodium
NC	nasal cannula
neg	negative
NG	nasogastric
NOI	nature of illness
NRB	nonrebreathing mask
NS	normal saline
NTG	nitroglycerin
N & V	nausea and vomiting
O_2	oxygen
OB	obstetrics
OBS	organic brain syndrome
OD	overdose
OTC	over-the-counter
$\overline{P}$	after

PCI	percutaneous coronary intervention
PCN	penicillin
PE	pulmonary embolism
PID	pelvic inflammatory disease
PO	by mouth
PMS	pulse, motor, sensation
prn	as needed
Pt	patient
PVC	premature ventricular contraction
Px	physical examination
q	every
Ⓡ	right
RBC	red blood count
REMCS	Regional Emergency Medical Communications System
RLQ	right lower quadrant
ROSC	return of spontaneous circulation
R/O	rule out
RSI	rapid sequence intubation
RTS	revised trauma score
RUQ	right upper quadrant
Rx	medication or prescription
$\bar{s}$	without
SC	subcutaneous
sec (s)	second
tab	tablet
temp	temperature
TIA	transient ischemic attack
tid	three times daily
TKO	to keep open
top	topical

continues

Tx	treatment
µg	microgram
UTI	urinary tract infection
VF	ventricular fibrillation
VS	vital signs
VT	ventricular tachycardia
WBC	white blood count
WPW	Wolff-Parkinson-White
w/	with
w/o	without
wk	week
wt	weight
yr	year

Communication Flipchart

Basic Directions

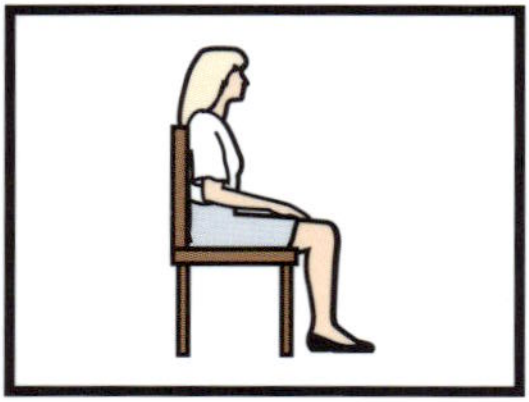

Sit down

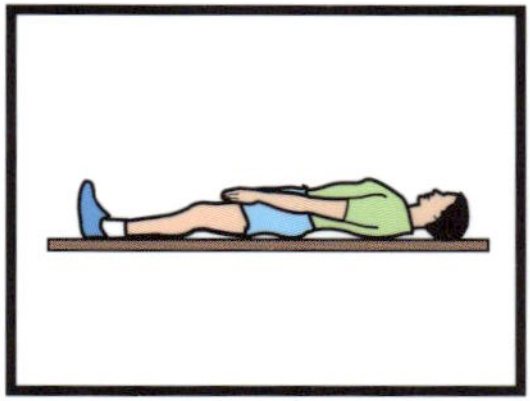

Lie down

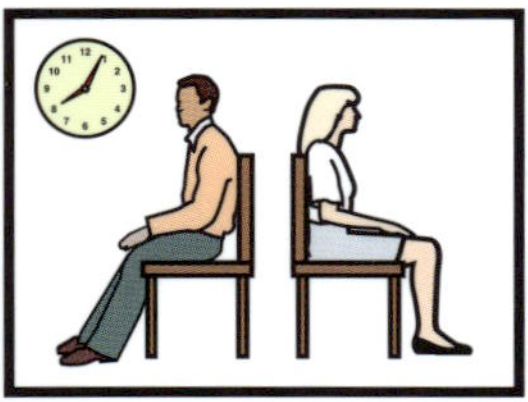

Wait

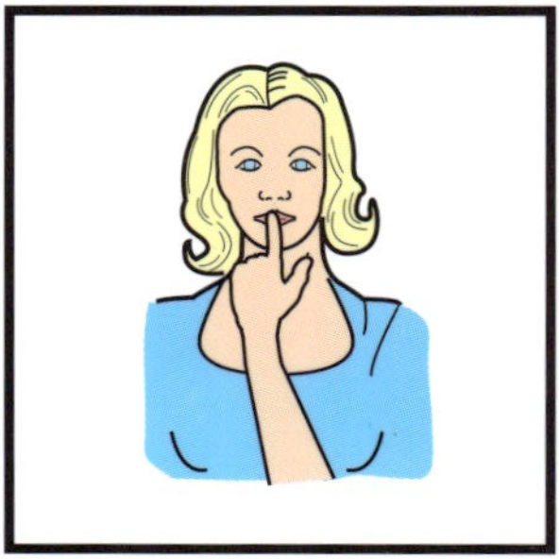

Quiet

Stop

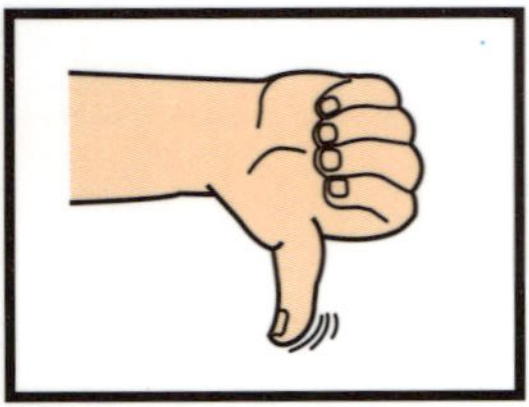

No

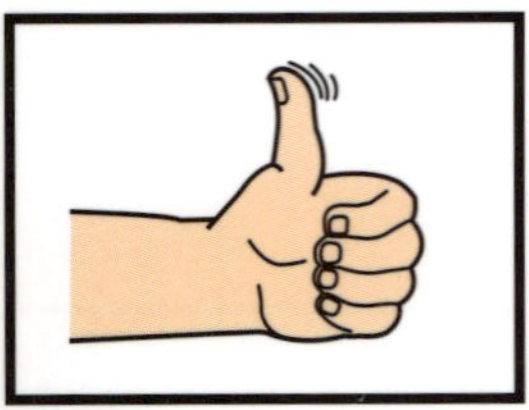

Yes

Identification

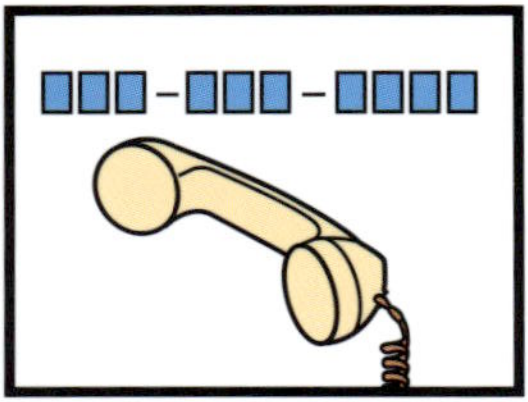

Phone

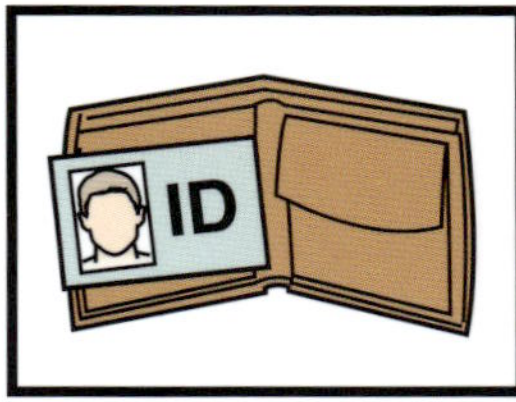

Name

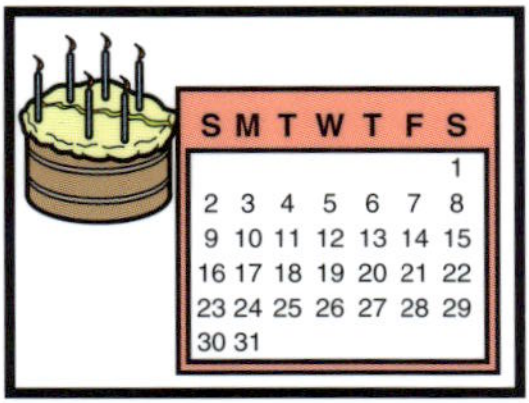

Date of Birth

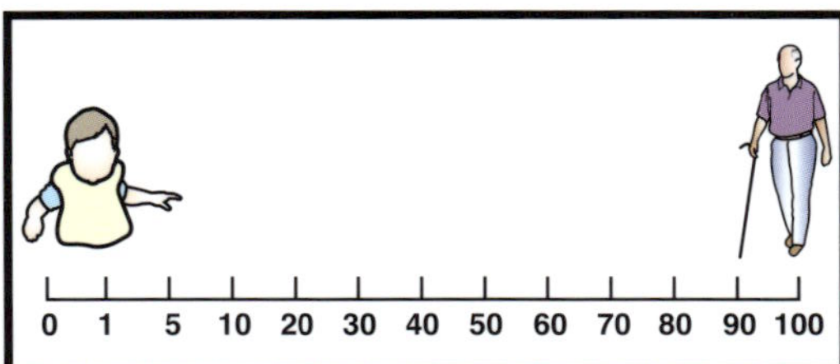

Age

A	B	C	D	E	F	G	H	I	J	K
L	M	N	O	P	Q	R	S	T	U	V
W	X	Y	Z							

Alphabet card

0	1	2	3	4	5	6	7	8	9

Number card

When

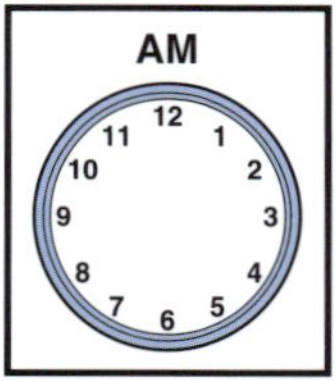

AM hours

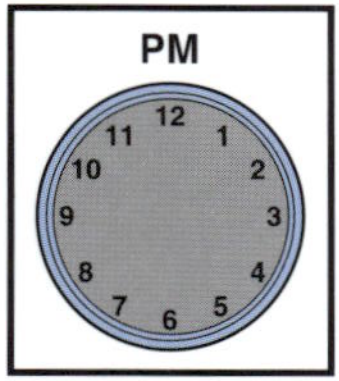

PM hours

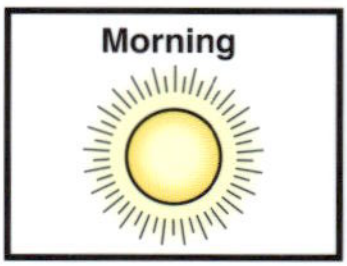

Day

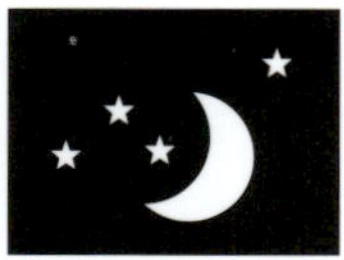

Night

Symptoms

Where does it hurt?

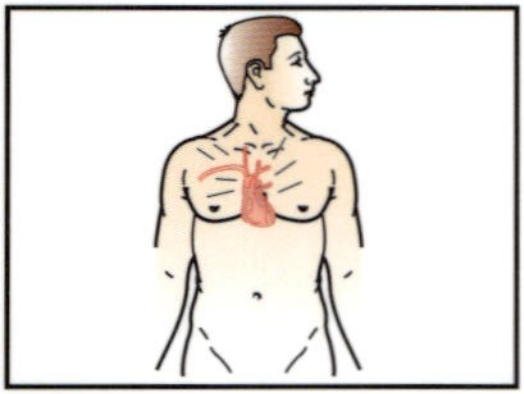

Chest pain

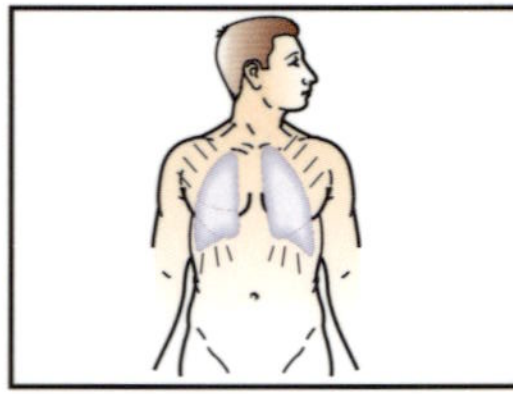

Respiratory distress

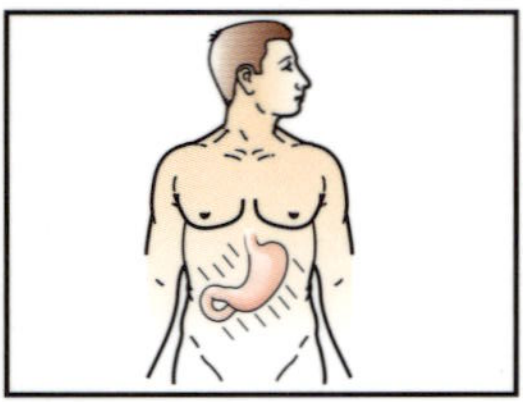

Stomach

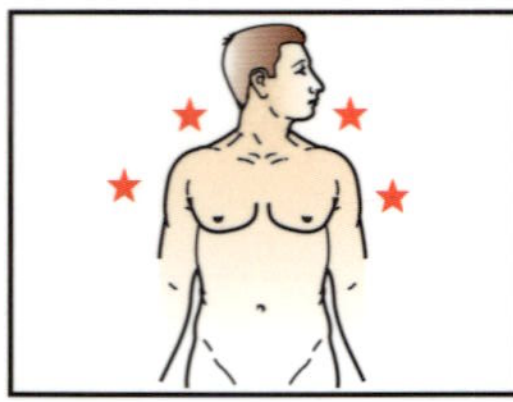

Muscle aches

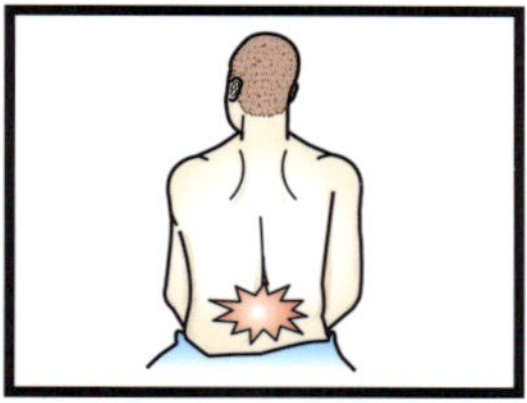

Backache

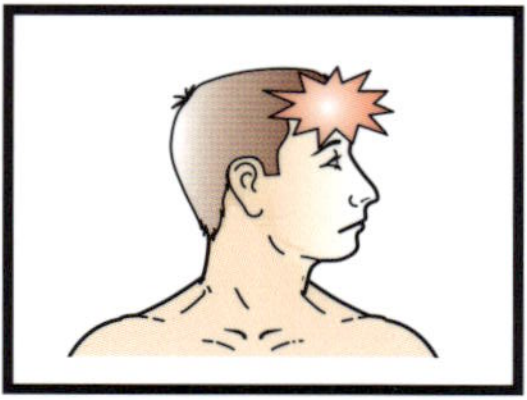

Headache

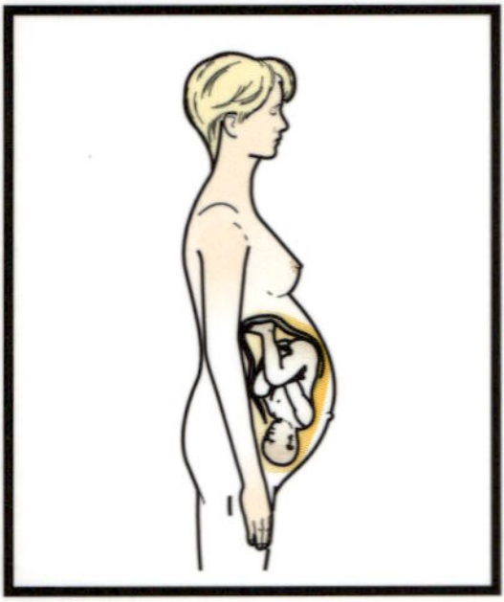

Pregnancy

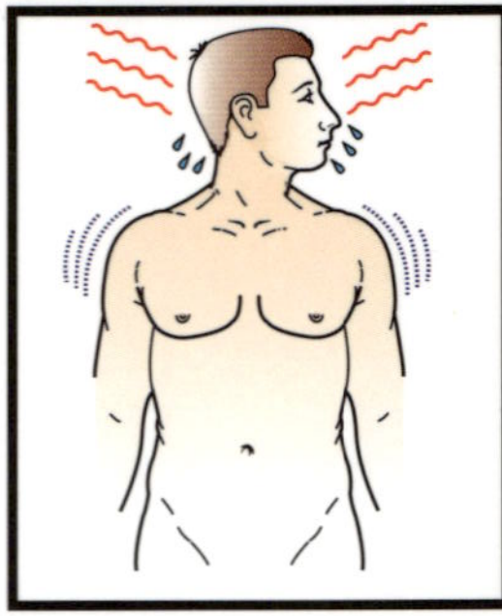

Fever/Chills

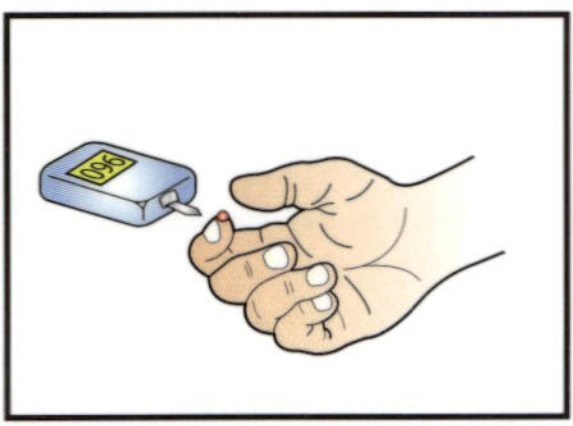

Diabetes

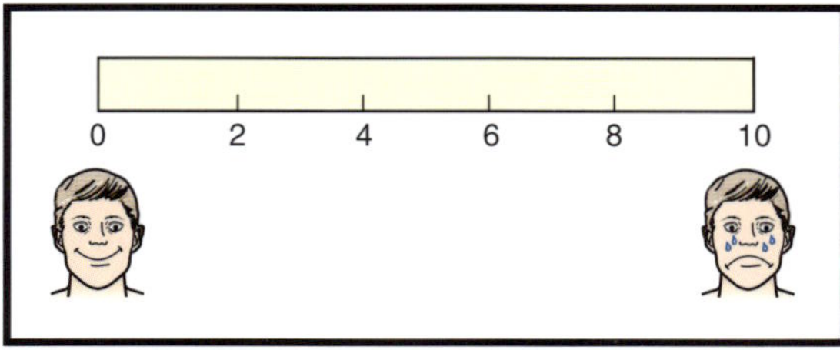

1–10 pain scale

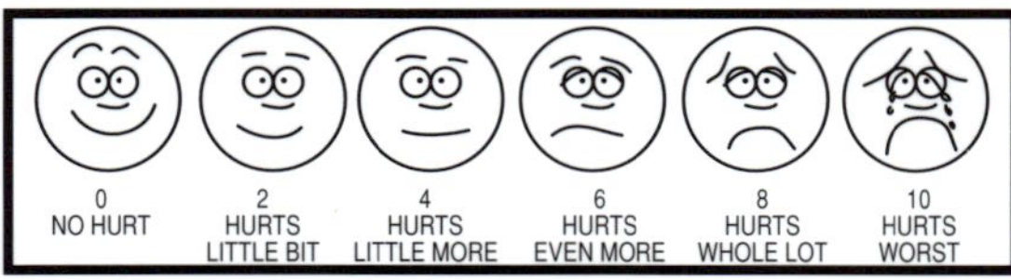

From Hockenberry MJ, Wilson D, Wikelstein ML. *Wong's Essentials of Pediatric Nursing,* ed. 7, St. Louis, 2005, p. 1259. Used with permission. Copyright, Mosby.

Intermittent pain

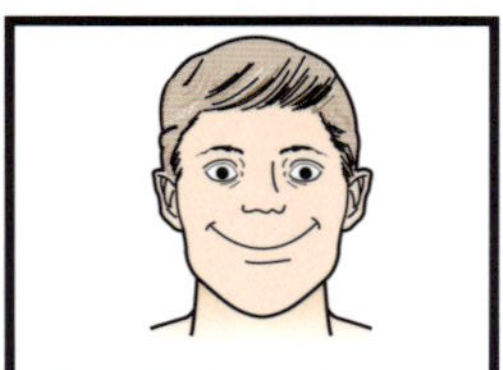

Better

Accidents

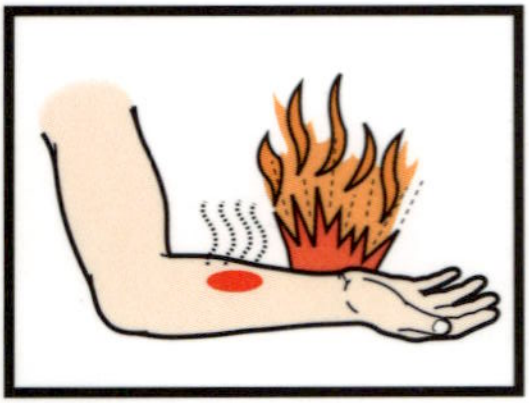

Burn

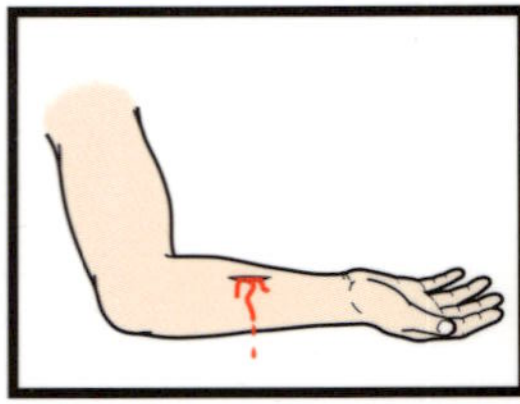

Cut

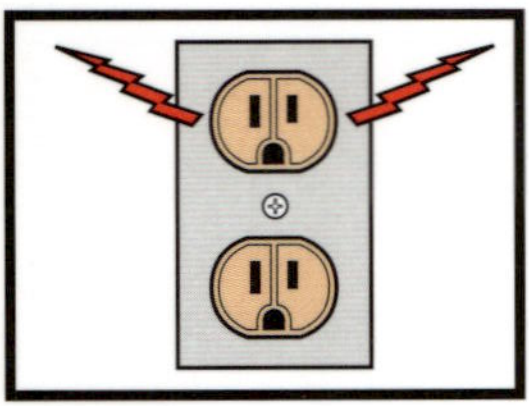

Electric outlet

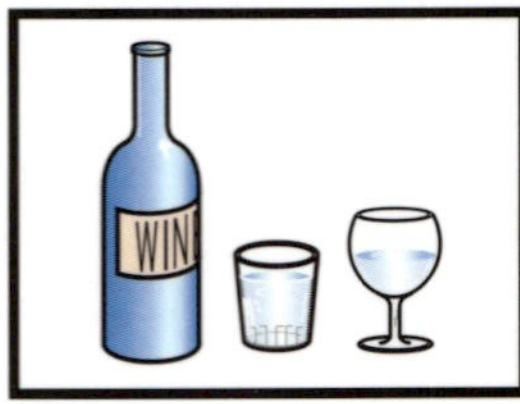

Alcohol

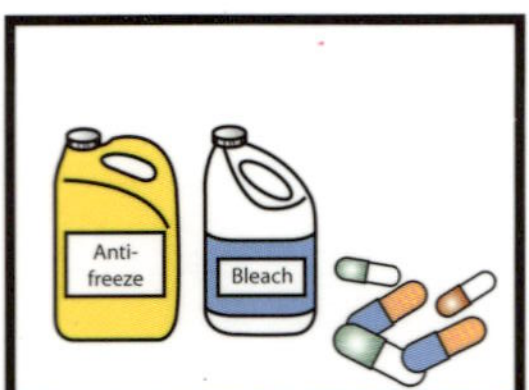

Poisons

Allergies

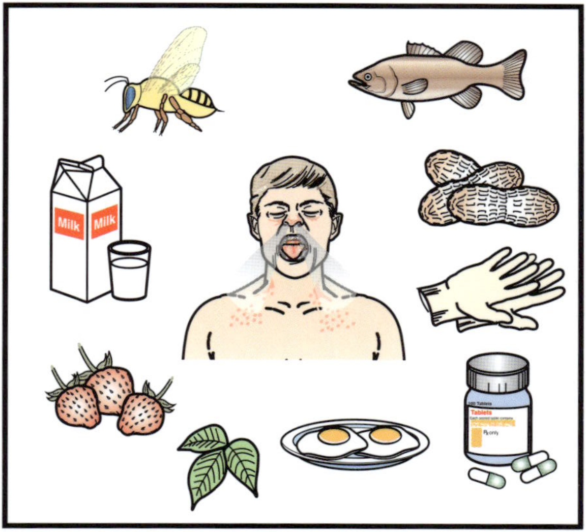

Allergies

Medications

Types

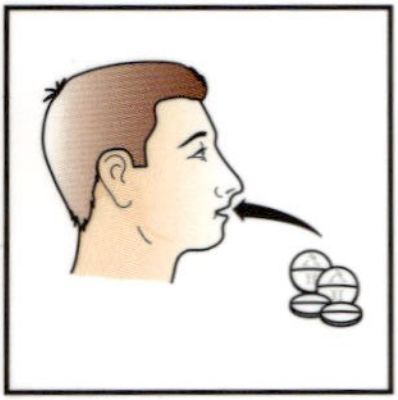

Oral

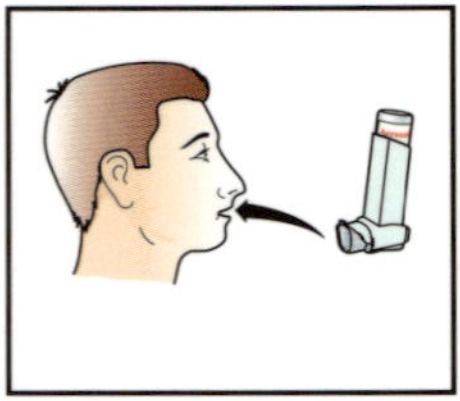

Inhaler

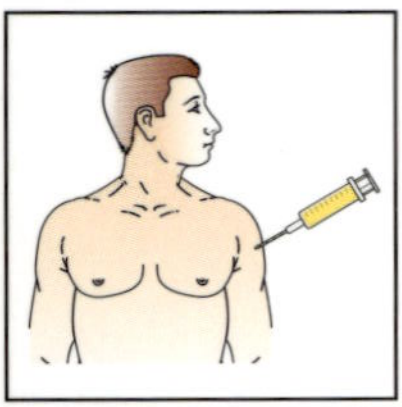

Needle

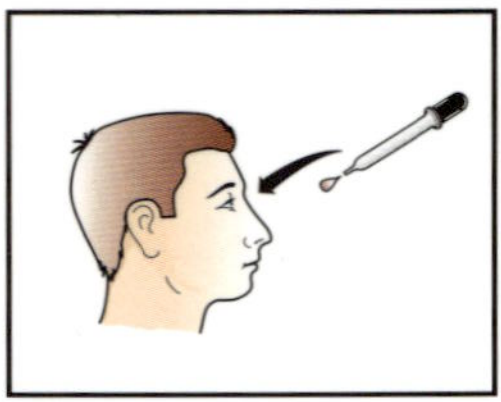

Dropper

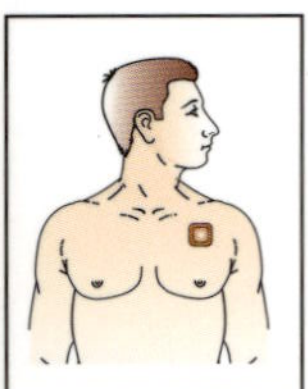

Patch

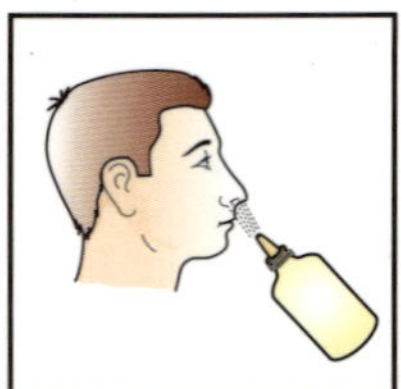

Nasal spray

Developmental Disabilities

Interventions for Patients with Challenging Behaviors

Individuals with developmental disabilities will present with varying physical and mental limitations. They may have difficulty communicating, learning, understanding, and responding to others. Human behavior is complex and unpredictable. Obvious and hidden disabilities can make interactions difficult.

Possible Indicators

- Look for a medical-alert bracelet, necklace, pocket card, shoelace tag
- Self-stimulation—hand-flapping, finger-flicking, body rocking or twirling, off-key humming, repetitive speech
- Repetition—sits up and down repeatedly, repeats sounds/mimics your words, twirls objects, handles objects compulsively, lines objects up in patterns
- Acclimation—wanders around looking at or touching objects, invades your personal space without warning
- Stands too close or too far away
- Resistant to physical contact
- Seems distracted or unaware
- Slow to answer—reacts more slowly to commands/requests
- Dissociated speech—reply with seemingly meaningless answers
- Unusual tone of voice—often a monotone quality or "robot voice," inappropriately loud or soft-spoken, interrupting or talking-over others, tone of voice does not demonstrate an appropriate level of fear or anger
- May not notice or understand nonverbal signs—body language, gestures, eye contact
- Lack of eye contact—may have little or no eye contact, may appear to be ignoring you or failing to pay attention

continues

- Unusual or awkward gait—toe-walking, unsteady gait, clumsy, difficulty balancing (especially when over-stimulated)
- Uncoordinated
- Explosive outbursts and temper tantrums
- Overreact to change in routine
- Reacts severely to sensory input—lights, sirens, voices, group situation
- Oblivious to danger/may resist rescue attempts
- May try to please you
  - Inclined to accept blame
  - Confess to any crime
  - Pretend to understand
  - May inaccurately answer yes/no questions
- Involvement in criminal activity
  - Frequent victims of crime
  - Frequently confess to crimes they didn't commit
  - More vulnerable to sexual assault and abuse
  - Oblivious to danger
  - Alternative sense of personal modesty
  - Gravitate to water/wandering
  - May resist rescue attempts
- May idolize authority figures
- Unusual facial features—flat nasal bridge, protruding tongue, short neck

During Encounters

- Seek out caregivers to help or provide advice
- Be safe—maintain safe distance

- Reduce distractions
  - Approach quietly
  - Stay back a few extra feet
  - Be aware that lights, sirens, fast-approaching vehicles may escalate crisis situation
  - Reduce stress/outside stimulation (less of everything)
  - Avoid crowding
- Be patient
- Use calm and reassuring tone of voice and slow hand gestures
- Stay at same level (don't tower over the person)
- Allow them to acclimate when possible
- Allow repetitive behaviors/self-stimulation unless they cause danger
- Ignore unwanted, inappropriate behaviors
- Model calm behavior and allow time for calming
- Don't expect or force eye contact or other "appropriate" body language
- Don't equate the inability to speak with deafness or illiteracy—pointing to pictures/symbols may help
- Use a normal volume and tone of voice
- Keep commands/questions brief, clear, and literal
- Explain, describe, and demonstrate what you are doing
- Avoid jargon, slang, and professional words
- Tell them what's next
- Allow extra time for responses
- Don't read meaning into their words
- Complete one topic at a time
- Dispel their fears
- Say "good job" to both kids and adults
- Recognize that they may have an altered sense of pain
- Document everything

Medical Precautions

- Frequent co-morbidities (seizures, hypertension, hearing impairment, physical disability, communication disorder)
- Be alert to positional asphyxia
  - Hypotonia
  - Support and constantly monitor breathing
- Altered sense of pain
- Adrenaline stays up (need extra time to cool/calm down)

Death of a Patient

Considerations

- Assess need for pastoral support.
- Contact the appropriate authorities.
- Stay with the body until the proper authorities arrive.
- Do not disturb or destroy potential evidence if a crime scene is suspected.

Assessment

- Form a general impression of the patient's condition.
- Establish responsiveness.
- Assess airway and breathing and confirm apnea.
- Assess pulselessness.
- If patient does not exhibit lividity and/or rigor mortis, begin resuscitative measures.
- If patient exhibits lividity and/or rigor mortis, contact medical command for pronouncement of death.
- Provide supportive measures to the family.
- If the patient is an infant and sudden infant death syndrome (SIDS) is suspected, provide the family with the telephone number for the New Jersey Sudden Infant Death Syndrome (SIDS) Center 1-800-545-7437. The SIDS Center provides culturally competent bereavement support for grieving families and SIDS risk-reduction education.
- Obtain patient history and reassess the environment.

Documentation

- Location of patient upon arrival
- Description of objects near the child upon arrival
- Unusual environmental conditions (i.e., high room temperature, abnormal odors, etc.)
- Presence of lividity or rigor mortis
- Consultation with medical command
- Complete Form A (www.state.nj.us/health/ems) if responding to unexplained death of an infant or child less than 3 years of age.

Unexplained Death of an Infant or Child Under 3 Years

Form A, available at **www.state.nj.us/health/ems**, is to be completed by the first team or individual(s) who respond to a sudden unexplained death of an infant or child less than 3 years of age. The lead emergency medical services and the lead law enforcement individuals are each expected to complete separate forms. Please indicate if information collected was obtained by interview or observation. Upon completion, forms are to be submitted to the medical examiner along with a copy of the patient care report, ambulance run sheet or police report, as applicable. Additional comments or notes should be provided on a separate sheet of paper labeled with the name, date of birth, and case number of the infant/child. Do not use the reverse side of any form.

Do Not Resuscitate Orders

Treatment

Withholding life support measures

↓

Life support may be withheld if any of the following exist: ①

- Patient qualifies for DNR status. ②
- Decapitation.
- Rigor mortis in a warm environment.
- Dependent lividity: venous pooling in dependent body parts.

↓

- Cover the body with a sheet.
- Contact the appropriate authorities.

↓

- Secure the scene.
- Do not remove personal property from the body.
- Do not disturb the scene or leave the body unattended.

continues

Treatment, continued

- Assess need for pastoral services for family/friends, if present.
- Activate pastoral support, as needed.

↓

- Complete your scene report.
- Relinquish scene control to the medical examiner or law enforcement.

Discontinuing resuscitative efforts in a traumatic cardiac arrest

↓

Follow the appropriate medical and cardiac protocols.

↓

Positive response to resuscitative measures.

- **No** → Contact medical command physician. Medical command may advise to discontinue efforts. → Follow medical command orders.
- **Yes** ↓

↓

- Transport ASAP.
- Continue resuscitation.

1. Contact medical command physician to discuss the case.
2. If the patient has a DNR form, ensure it has been signed by the patient/surrogate.

Heat Index

Temperature (˚F)

Relative Humidity (%)	80	82	84	86	88	90	92	94	96	98	100	102	104	106	108	110
40	80	81	83	85	88	91	94	97	101	105	109	114	119	124	130	136
45	80	82	84	87	89	93	96	100	104	109	114	119	124	130	137	
50	81	83	85	88	91	95	99	103	108	113	118	124	131	137		
55	81	84	86	89	93	97	101	106	112	117	124	130	137			
60	82	84	88	91	95	100	105	110	116	123	129	137				
65	82	85	89	93	98	103	108	114	121	128	136					
70	83	86	90	95	100	105	112	119	126	134						
75	84	88	92	97	103	109	116	124	132							
80	84	89	94	100	106	113	121	129								
85	85	90	96	102	110	117	126	135								
90	86	91	98	105	113	122	131									
95	86	93	100	108	117	127										
100	87	95	103	112	121	132										

Likelihood of heat disorders with prolonged exposure or strenuous activity:

Caution   Extreme caution   Danger   Extreme danger

Reprinted from: US National Weather Service. Available at: http://www.nws.noaa.gov/om/heat/index_shtml. Accessed October 2010.

Wind Chill Chart

Wind (mph)	Temperature (°F)																	
Calm	40	35	30	25	20	15	10	5	0	-5	-10	-15	-20	-25	-30	-35	-40	-45
5	36	31	25	19	13	7	1	-5	-11	-16	-22	-28	-34	-40	-46	-52	-57	-63
10	34	27	21	15	9	3	-4	-10	-16	-22	-28	-35	-41	-47	-53	-59	-66	-72
15	32	25	19	13	6	0	-7	-13	-19	-26	-32	-39	-45	-51	-58	-64	-71	-77
20	30	24	17	11	4	-2	-9	-15	-22	-29	-35	-42	-48	-55	-61	-68	-74	-81
25	29	23	16	9	3	-4	-11	-17	-24	-31	-37	-44	-51	-58	-64	-71	-78	-84
30	28	22	15	8	1	-5	-12	-19	-26	-33	-39	-46	-53	-60	-67	-73	-80	-87
35	28	21	14	7	0	-7	-14	-21	-27	-34	-41	-48	-55	-62	-69	-76	-82	-89
40	27	20	13	6	-1	-8	-15	-22	-29	-36	-43	-50	-57	-64	-71	-78	-84	-91
45	26	19	12	5	-2	-9	-16	-23	-30	-37	-44	-51	-58	-65	-72	-79	-86	-93
50	26	19	12	4	-3	-10	-17	-24	-31	-38	-45	-52	-60	-67	-74	-81	-88	-95
55	25	18	11	4	-3	-11	-18	-25	-32	-39	-46	-54	-61	-68	-75	-82	-89	-97
60	25	17	10	3	-4	-11	-19	-26	-33	-40	-48	-55	-62	-69	-76	-84	-91	-98

Frostbite Times: 30 minutes / 10 minutes / 5 minutes

$$\text{Wind Chill (°F)} = 35.74 + 0.6215T - 35.75(V^{0.16}) + 0.4275T(V^{0.16})$$

Where, T= Air Temperature (°F) V= Wind Speed (mph)

Effective 11/01/01

Courtesy of NWS/NOAA. Available from: www.weather.gov/os/windchill/index/shtml.

Measurement Conversions

Conversion Formulas

To convert from the unit of measure in Column B to the unit of measure in Column C, multiply the number of units in Column B by the multiplier in Column A. To convert from Column C to B, use the multiplier in Column D.

A	B	C	D
0.3937	Centimeter (cm)	Inch (in)	2.54
10	Centimeter (cm)	Millimeter (mm)	0.1
0.3048	Feet	Meters	3.281
25.4	Inches (in)	Millimeters (mm)	0.394
1000	Milligram (mg)	Microgram (mcg)	0.001
1000	Liter (L)	Milliliters (mL) or cubic centimeters (cc)	0.001
F – 32) × 5/9	Fahrenheit (F)	Celsius (C)	C × 9/5 + 32
0.4536	Pounds (lb)	Kilograms (kg)	2.205

Adult Height, Weight, Temperature Conversions

HEIGHT			WEIGHT		TEMPERATURE	
ft/in	in	cm	lb	kg	F	C
4'8"	56	142	90	40.9	212	100 (boiling point)
4'9"	57	145	100	45.5	108	42.2
5'0"	58	147	110	50.0	107	41.6
5'1"	59	150	120	54.5	106	41.1
5'2"	60	152	130	59.1	105	40.6

5′3″	61	155	140	63.6	104	40.0
5′4″	62	157	150	68.2	103	39.4
5′5″	63	160	160	72.7	102	38.9
5′6″	64	163	170	77.3	101	38.3
5′7″	65	165	180	81.8	100	37.8
5′8″	66	168	190	86.4	99	37.2
5′9″	67	170	200	90.9	98.6	37.0
6′0″	68	173	210	95.5	98	36.7
6′1″	69	175	225	102.3	97	36.1
6′2″	70	178	250	113.6	96	35.6
6′3″	71	180	275	125.0	95	35.0
6′4″	72	183	300	136.4	94	34.4
6′5″	73	185			93	34.0
6′6″	74	188			92	33.3
6′7″	75	191			91	32.8
6′8″	76	193			90	32.1
6′9″	77	196			32	0 (freezing)

Medical Spanish

General

Hello.	Hola.
My name is . . .	Me llamo . . .
Yes	Sí
No	No
Please	Por favor
Thank you	Gracias
What is your name?	¿Cómo se llama usted?
Identification	Identificación
I am going to help you.	Estoy aquí para ayudarle.
I need to examine you.	Necesito examinarlo(la)*
Answer yes or no.	Responda sí o no.
Do you understand?	¿Comprende?
I don't understand.	No comprendo.
One	Uno
Two	Dos
Three	Tres
Four	Quatro
Five	Cinco
Six	Seis
Seven	Siete
Eight	Ocho
Nine	Nueve
Ten	Diez

*"lo" and "la" are direct object pronouns meaning "you," "him," or "her" (lo = masculine, la = feminine).

Trauma

Are you hurt?	¿Está herido?
How did it happen?	¿Cómo occurió?
Did you fall?	¿Se cayó?
How far did you fall?	¿De qué altura se cayó?
Did you lose consciousness?	¿Perdio el conocimiento?
Are you bleeding?	¿Está sangrando?

Pain

Point to where it hurts.	Señale dónde le duele.
Does this hurt?	¿Le duele esto?
Is the pain strong or weak?	¿Es el dolor fuerto o débil?*
Unbearable	Insoportable
Hurts a lot	Duele mucho
Hurts	Duele
Hurts a little	Duele un poquito
No pain	No duele
Sharp	Agudo
Dull	No tan agudo
Crushing	Aplastante
Tight	Apretado
When did it start?	¿Cuándo empezó?
half hour	media hora
1 hour	una hora
2 hours	dos horas
3 hours	tres horas
Longer than 3 hours	Más de tres horas
1 day ago	Ayer

*Leve, débil, and suave can all be used to describe a weak or a slight pain.

Pregnancy

Are you pregnant?	¿Está embarazada?
Are you having contractions?	¿Tiene contracciones?
How many minutes between contractions?	¿Cuántos minutos entre las contracciones?

Medical

Are you sick?	¿Está enfermo?
Are you having trouble breathing?	¿Tiene problemas para respirar?
Do you have allergies?	¿Tiene alergias?
When did you last eat?	¿Cuándo fue su última comida?
Morning	En la mañana
Afternoon	En la tarde
Evening	En la noche
What is making you sick?	¿Qué le hace sentirse mal?
Something you ate or drank	Algo que comió o tomó
Something that contacted your skin	Algo que entró en contacto con su piel
Something you injected	Algo que se inyectó
Something you inhaled	Algo que inhaló
Do you have asthma?	¿Tiene asma?

Medications

Do you take medicine every day?	¿Toma medicamentos diariamente?
What medicine do you take?	¿Qué medicamentos toma?
Heart	El corazón
Diabetes	La diabetes
Stroke	Derrame cerebral
Asthma	El asma
Emphysema	Enfisema
Stomach	El estómago
Bee stings	La picadura de abeja
Pregnancy	El embarazo

Where is the medicine?	¿Dónde está el medicamento?
When did you take it?	¿Cuándo lo tomó?
Morning	En la mañana
Afternoon	En la tarde
Evening	En la noche
How much did you take?	¿Cuánto tomó?
Less than half	Menos de la mitad
More than half	Más de la mitad
Do you have allergies to medicines?	¿Tiene alergias a alguna medicina?
Penicillin	Penicilina
Codeine	Codeína
Morphine	Morphina
Sulfa	Sulfa
Aspirin	Aspirina
Lidocaine	Lidocaína

Treatment

We are going to take care of you.	Nosotros vamos a atenderlo.
We're going to the hospital.	Vamos al hospital.
Take several deep breaths so I can listen to you breathe.	Respire profundo varias veces para que yo pueda escucharlo respirar
I am going to give you some oxygen.	Le voy a dar un poco de oxígeno.
I am going to give you some medicine to help you.	Le voy a dar un medicamento para ayudarlo.
Lay in the position that is comfortable for you.	Acúestese en una posición que se sienta cómodo.
We are going to put a safety collar around your neck so your head does not move.	Le vamos a poner un collarin ortopédico alrededor del cuello para immovilizarle la cabeza.
Try not to move.	No se mueva.

Medications

Routes of Administration

TABLE 1 Routes of Administration: Words and Their Meanings

This Word ...	From These Latin Words ...	Means
Inhalation	*Inhalatio* (drawing air into the lungs)	Inhaling or breathing in
Intramuscular (IM)	*Intra* (into) and *muscularis* (of the muscles)	Into muscle
Intraosseous (IO)	*Intra* (into) and *osse* (bone)	Into bone
Intravenous (IV)	*Intra* (into) and *venosus* (of the veins)	Into vein
Per os (PO)	*Per* (by) and *os* (mouth)	By mouth
Per rectum (PR)	*Per* (by) and *rectum* (rectum)	By rectum
Subcutaneous (SC)	*Sub* (under) and *cutis* (skin)	Under the skin
Sublingual (SL)	*Sub* (under) and *lingua* (relating to the tongue)	Under the tongue
Transcutaneous (transdermal)	*Trans* (through) and *cutis* (skin)	Through the skin
Intranasal (IN)	*Intra* (into) and *nasal* (nose)	Into the nose

Medications and Their Uses

Trade names start with an uppercase letter and appear in **blue**. **Generic names** start with a lowercase letter and appear in **red**. The primary type of medical problem for which the medication is used is listed, and the type of medication is shown in parentheses, when indicated. **Noting patients' medications can help the responder determine the types of medical problems patients may have, even if they are unsure of their history or are unconscious.**

Medication	Use
Abilify	Bipolar disorder, schizophrenia
Accolate	Asthma
Accupril	High blood pressure, congestive heart failure
acetaminophen with codeine	Pain
Aciphex	Gastric problems (antiulcer)
Actiq	Pain (narcotic analgesic)
Actonel	Osteoporosis
Actos	Diabetes (oral antidiabetic)
acyclovir	Viral infections (antiviral)
Adderall	Attention deficit/hyperactivity disorder
Adipex	Weight loss
Advair	Breathing problems
albuterol	Breathing problems (bronchodilator)
Aldactazide	High blood pressure (diuretic/water pill)
Aldactone	Congestive heart failure (diuretic/water pill)
Aldomet	High blood pressure
alendronate	Osteoporosis
Alesse 28	Birth control pills
Allegra	Allergies (antihistamine)
Alli	Weight loss
allopurinol	Gout, kidney stones
alprazolam	Anxiety, depression (sedative/antianxiety)
Altace	High blood pressure (ACE inhibitor)

continues

Alupent	Asthma, breathing problems (bronchodilator)
Amaryl	Diabetes (oral antidiabetic)
Ambien	Insomnia (hypnotic)
Amitiza	Gastrointestinal problems
amitriptyline	Depression (antidepressant)
amlodipine	High blood pressure, angina
amoxicillin	Infection (antibiotic)
Amoxil	Infection (antibiotic)
Anaprox	Arthritis (anti-inflammatory)
Ansaid	Arthritis (anti-inflammatory)
Antivert	Dizziness, motion sickness (antivertigo)
Apresoline	High blood pressure (antihypertensive)
Aricept	Alzheimer's disease
Artane	Parkinson's disease (anti-Parkinson)
Arthrotec	Arthritis (anti-inflammatory)
Asacol	Ulcerative colitis (antibacterial)
Asmanex	Asthma (anti-inflammatory)
Aspirin	Analgesic
Atarax	Anxiety, behavioral disorders (sedative)
atenolol	High blood pressure, heart problems, angina (beta blocker)
Ativan	Anxiety (sedative/antianxiety)
Atrovent	Breathing problems (bronchodilator)
Augmentin	Infection (antibiotic)
Avandamet	Diabetes
Avandia	Diabetes (oral antidiabetic)
Avapro	High blood pressure
Avodart	Prostate enlargement
Axid	Ulcers (antiulcer)
azithromycin	Infection (antibiotic)
Azulfidine	Ulcerative colitis (antibacterial)

Bactrim	Infection (antibiotic)
Bactroban	Impetigo (antibiotic)
Benadryl	Allergies (antihistamine)
benazepril	High blood pressure, congestive heart failure
Benicar	High blood pressure
Bentyl	Irritable bowel syndrome (anticholinergic)
benzonatate	Cough (antitussive)
Biaxin	Infection (antibiotic)
bisoprolol	High blood pressure (diuretic)
Boniva	Osteoporosis
Brethine	Asthma, breathing problems (bronchodilator)
Bumex	Edema, congestive heart failure (diuretic)
bupropion	Depression, smoking cessation
BuSpar	Anxiety (antianxiety)
buspirone	Anxiety (antianxiety)
Byetta	Diabetes
Caduet	High blood pressure
Calan	Angina, high blood pressure, rapid heart rate
Capoten	High blood pressure, congestive heart failure
captopril	High blood pressure, congestive heart failure
Carafate	Ulcers (antiulcer)
carbamazepine	Seizure disorder (anticonvulsant)
Cardizem	Heart problems, angina (coronary vasodilator)
Cardura	High blood pressure (alpha blocker)
carisoprodol	Muscle spasms (muscle relaxant)
Cartia	Angina, heart problems (calcium-channel blocker)
carvedilol	High blood pressure
Catapres	High blood pressure (antihypertensive)

continues

Ceclor	Infection (antibiotic)
cefaclor	Infection (antibiotic)
cefdinir	Infection (antibiotic)
cefixime	Infection (antibiotic)
cefprozil	Infection (antibiotic)
Ceftin	Infection (antibiotic)
cefuroxime	Infection (antibiotic)
Cefzil	Infection (antibiotic)
Celebrex	Arthritis (anti-inflammatory)
Celexa	Depression (antidepressant)
cephalexin	Infection (antibiotic)
cetirizine	Antihistamine
Chantix	Smoking cessation
Cialis	Male impotence
Ciloxin	Infection (antibiotic)
cimetidine	Ulcers, gastric problems (antiulcer)
Cipro	Infection (antibiotic)
citalopram	Depression
Clarinex	Allergies (antihistamine)
Claritin	Allergies (antihistamine)
clarithromycin	Infection (antibiotic)
clindamycin	Infection (antibiotic)
Clinoril	Arthritis pain (anti-inflammatory)
clonazepam	Seizure disorder (anticonvulsant)
clonidine	High blood pressure (antihypertensive)
clopidogrel	Antiplatelet
clotrimazole	Fungal infection (antifungal)
Colestid	High cholesterol (cholesterol-lowering agent)
Combivent	Breathing problems (bronchodilator)
Compazine	Nausea (antiemetic)

Concerta	Attention deficit/hyperactivity disorder
Coreg	High blood pressure, heart problems
Corgard	Heart problems, angina (beta blocker)
Cotrim	Infection (anti-infective)
Coumadin	Blood clots (blood thinner)
Cozaar	High blood pressure
Crestor	High cholesterol
cyclobenzaprine	Muscle spasms (muscle relaxant)
Cymbalta	Depression
Darvocet-N	Pain management (narcotic analgesic)
Daypro	Arthritis (anti-inflammatory)
Deltasone	Severe inflammation (anti-inflammatory)
Demadex	Edema, congestive heart failure (diuretic)
Demerol	Pain (narcotic analgesic)
Depakote	Seizure disorder (anticonvulsant)
Desyrel	Depression (antidepressant)
Detrol	Overactive bladder
Dexedrine	Narcolepsy, attention-deficit disorder
dexmethylphenidate	Attention deficit/hyperactivity disorder
DiaBeta	Diabetes (oral antidiabetic)
Diabinese	Diabetes (oral antidiabetic)
diazepam	Anxiety (antianxiety)
diclofenac	Inflammation (anti-inflammatory)
Diflucan	Fungal infection (antifungal)
Digitek	Heart problems
digoxin	Heart problems
Dilantin	Seizure disorder (anticonvulsant)
diltiazem	Heart problems, angina (coronary vasodilator)
Diovan	High blood pressure (antihypertensive)
Dipentum	Ulcerative colitis

continues

diphenhydramine	Allergies (antihistamine)
dipyridamole	Thromboembolism
Ditropan	Bladder problems (antispasmodic)
Donnatal	Irritable bowel syndrome (anticholinergic)
doxazosin	Hypertension, prostate problems
doxycycline	Infection (antibiotic)
Duricef	Infection (antibiotic)
Dyazide	High blood pressure, edema (diuretic)
DynaCirc	High blood pressure
E.E.S.	Infection (antibiotic)
Effexor	Depression (antidepressant)
Elavil	Depression (antidepressant)
Eldepryl	Parkinson's disease (anti-Parkinson)
Elocon	Dermatologic problems
Emend	Nausea (antiemetic)
enalapril	High blood pressure, heart failure
Enbrel	Rheumatoid arthritis
E-Mycin	Infection (antibiotic)
Entex	Cough and congestion (expectorant)
epinephrine	Cardiac arrest, allergic reactions (antihistamine)
Epivir	Antiretroviral
Ery-Tab	Infection (antibiotic)
erythromycin	Infection (antibiotic)
escitalopram	Depression
Esidrix	High blood pressure (diuretic/water pill)
Eskalith	Behavioral disorders (antimanic)
Estrace	Estrogen therapy
Estraderm	Estrogen therapy
estradiol	Menopause, gynecologic problems
etodolac	Arthritis, pain (anti-inflammatory)
Evista	Osteoporosis

famotidine	Ulcers, gastric problems (antiulcer)
Feldene	Arthritis (anti-inflammatory)
fentanyl	Pain management (narcotic analgesic)
finasteride	Prostate enlargement
Fiorinal	Pain management (non-narcotic analgesic)
Flagyl	Infections (antibacterial)
Flexeril	Muscle spasms (muscle relaxant)
flexofenadine	Antihistamine
Flomax	Enlarged prostate (alpha blocker)
Flonase	Allergies
Flovent	Breathing problems
Floxin	Infection (antibiotic)
fluconazole	Fungal infection
fluoxetine	Depression (antidepressant)
flurbiprofen	Inflammation (anti-inflammatory)
folic acid	Anemia
Fosamax	Osteoporosis
fosinopril	Osteoporosis
furosemide	Congestive heart failure (diuretic/water pill)
gabapentin	Seizures
Gabitril	Seizure disorder (antiseizure)
Gantrisin	Infection (antibiotic)
gemfibrozil	High cholesterol (cholesterol-lowering agent)
Geodon	Antipsychotic
glimepiride	Diabetes (hyperglycemia)
glipizide	Diabetes (oral antidiabetic)
Glucophage	Diabetes (oral antidiabetic)
Glucotrol	Diabetes (oral antidiabetic)
Glucovance	Diabetes (oral antidiabetic)
glyburide	Diabetes (oral hypoglycemic)

continues

Glycolax	Constipation
granisetron	Nausea
guaifenesin	Cough and congestion (expectorant)
Halcion	Insomnia (hypnotic/sedative)
Haldol	Psychotic disorders (antipsychotic)
HCTZ	High blood pressure (diuretic/water pill)
Humira	Rheumatoid arthritis
Humulin	Diabetes (insulin)
hydrochlorothiazide	High blood pressure (diuretic)
hydrocodone	Cough, pain (narcotic)
HydroDiuril	High blood pressure (diuretic/water pill)
hydroxyzine	Anxiety, behavioral disorders (sedative)
Hygroton	High blood pressure (diuretic/water pill)
Hytrin	High blood pressure (alpha blocker)
Hyzaar	High blood pressure (antihypertensive)
ibuprofen	Inflammation, pain, fever (anti-inflammatory)
Imdur	Heart problems, angina (coronary vasodilator)
Imitrex	Migraine headaches (antimigraine)
Inderal	High blood pressure, heart problems, angina (beta blocker)
Indocin	Osteoarthritis, pain (anti-inflammatory)
indomethacin	Arthritis (anti-inflammatory)
Intal	Asthma (mast cell stabilizer)
Iophen	Cough (antitussive)
Isoptin	Angina, high blood pressure, rapid heart rate
Isordil	Heart problems, angina (coronary vasodilator)
isosorbide dinitrate	Heart problems, angina (coronary vasodilator)

K-Dur	Potassium replacement, taken with diuretics
K-Tab	Potassium replacement, taken with diuretics
Keflex	Infection (antibiotic)
Keppra	Seizure disorder (anticonvulsant)
ketoconazole	Fungal infection (antifungal)
ketorolac	Pain management (anti-inflammatory)
Klonopin	Seizure disorder (anticonvulsant)
labetalol	High blood pressure (beta blocker)
Lamictal	Seizure disorder (anti-epileptic)
Lamisil	Antifungal
Lanoxin	Heart problems
Lasix	Congestive heart failure (diuretic/water pill)
Lescol	High cholesterol (cholesterol-lowering agent)
Levaquin	Infection (antibiotic)
Levitra	Male impotence
Levothroid	Thyroid disease (thyroid hormone)
levothyroxine	Thyroid problems (thyroid hormone)
Levoxyl	Thyroid disease (thyroid hormone)
Lexapro	Depression
Librax	Peptic ulcer (anticholinergic)
Lipitor	High cholesterol (cholesterol-lowering agent)
lisinopril	High blood pressure
lithium carbonate	Behavioral disorders (antipsychotic)
Lodine	Arthritis, pain (anti-inflammatory)
Loestrin Fe	Birth control pills
Lomotil	Diarrhea (antidiarrheal)
Lopid	High cholesterol (cholesterol-lowering agent)
Lopressor	High blood pressure (beta blocker)

continues

Lorabid	Infection (antibiotic)
loracarbef	Infection (antibiotic)
loratadine	Allergies (antihistamine)
lorazepam	Anxiety (sedative/antianxiety)
Lorcet	Pain (narcotic analgesic)
Lortab	Pain (narcotic analgesic)
Lotensin	High blood pressure (ACE inhibitor)
Lotrel	Hypertension
Lotrimin	Fungal infection (antifungal cream and ointment)
Lotrisone	Fungal infection (antifungal cream)
lovastatin	High cholesterol (cholesterol-lowering agent)
Lozol	Congestive heart failure, high blood pressure
Lunesta	Sleep aid
Luvox	Parkinson's disease (anti-Parkinson)
Lyrica	Nerve pain
Macrobid	Urinary tract infection (antibiotic)
Macrodantin	Urinary tract infection (antibiotic)
marijuana	Comfort management
Maxzide	High blood pressure (diuretic/water pill)
meclizine	Dizziness, vertigo, motion sickness (antiemetic)
medroxyprogesterone	Gynecologic problems
meloxicam	Inflammation, pain
metformin	Diabetes
methadone	Pain (narcotic analgesic), opiate withdrawal
methylphenidate	Attention deficit disorder, narcolepsy
methylprednisolone	Anti-inflammatory
metoclopromide	Gastric problems (antiemetic)
metoprolol tartrate	High blood pressure, heart problems (beta blocker)

metronidazole	Infection (anti-infective)
Mevacor	High cholesterol (cholesterol-lowering agent)
Micro-K	Potassium replacement, taken with diuretics
Micronase	Diabetes (oral antidiabetic)
Minipress	High blood pressure (antihypertensive)
Minocin	Infection (antibiotic)
minocycline	Infection (antibiotic)
Miralax	Constipation
Mirapex	Parkinson's disease (anti-Parkinson)
Mircette	Birth control pills
mirtazapine	Anxiety, depression
Mobic	Inflammation, pain
moexipril	High blood pressure
Monopril	High blood pressure
morphine	Pain management (narcotic analgesic)
Motrin	Inflammation, pain, fever (anti-inflammatory)
nabumetone	Inflammation, pain (anti-inflammatory)
Namenda	Alzheimer's disease
Naprosyn	Inflammation, pain (anti-inflammatory)
naproxen	Inflammation, pain (anti-inflammatory)
Nasacort	Asthma, breathing problems (anti-inflammatory)
Nasonex	Allergies (anti-inflammatory)
Necon	Birth control pills
Neurontin	Seizure disorders (anticonvulsant)
Nexium	Gastric problems
Niaspan	High cholesterol
nifedipine	Heart problems, angina (coronary vasodilator)

continues

Nitro-Dur	Heart problems, angina (coronary vasodilator)
nitrofurantoin	Urinary tract infection
nitroglycerin	Heart problems, angina (coronary vasodilator)
Nitrostat	Heart problems, angina (coronary vasodilator)
nizatidine	Ulcers (antiulcer)
Nizoral	Fungal infection (antifungal)
Norco	Pain (narcotic analgesic)
Normodyne	High blood pressure
nortriptyline	Depression (antidepressant)
Norvasc	High blood pressure (calcium-channel blocker)
nystatin	Fungal infection (antifungal)
omeprazole	Ulcers, gastric problems (antiulcer)
Omnicef	Infections (antibiotic)
Omnipen	Infections (antibiotic)
ondansetron	Nausea
Ortho-Cept	Birth control pills
Ortho-Cyclen	Birth control pills
Ortho-Novum	Birth control pills
Ortho Tri-Cyclen	Birth control pills
Oruvail	Arthritis pain (anti-inflammatory)
oseltamivir	Antiviral
oxaprozin	Inflammation, pain, fever (anti-inflammatory)
oxcarbazepine	Seizures
oxybutynin	Bladder problems (antispasmodic)
oxycodone	Pain (narcotic analgesic)
Oxy-Contin	Pain (narcotic analgesic)
Pamelor	Depression (antidepressant)

pantoprazole	Gastric problems, ulcers
paroxetine	Depression (antidepressant)
Pataday	Allergies (antihistamine)
Patanol	Allergies (antihistamine)
Paxil	Depression (antidepressant)
Pediazole	Infection (antibiotic)
penicillin	Infection (antibiotic)
pentoxifylline	Vascular disease (blood thinner)
Pepcid	Ulcers, gastric problems (antiulcer)
Percocet	Pain (narcotic analgesic)
Percodan	Pain (narcotic analgesic)
Persantine	Thromboembolism
phenazopyridine	Urinary tract irritation, infection
Phenergan	Nausea (antiemetic)
phenobarbital	Seizure disorder (anticonvulsant)
phentermine	Weight loss
phenytoin	Seizure disorder (anticonvulsant)
Plavix	Thromboembolism (antiplatelet)
Plendil	High blood pressure (calcium-channel blocker)
potassium chloride	Potassium replacement, taken with diuretics
Prandin	Diabetes (oral antidiabetic)
Pravachol	High cholesterol (cholesterol-lowering agent)
prednisone	Severe inflammation (anti-inflammatory)
Premarin	Menopause, gynecologic problems (estrogen)
Prempro	Menopause, gynecological problems
Prevacid	Ulcers, gastric problems (antiulcer)
Prilosec	Ulcers, gastric problems (antiulcer)
Prinivil	High blood pressure (ACE inhibitor)

continues

Pro-Banthine	Peptic ulcer (anticholinergic)
Procan	Rapid heart rate, tachycardia (antiarrhythmic)
Procardia	Heart problems, angina (coronary vasodilator)
Proloprim	Infection, mainly urinary tract (antibiotic)
promethazine	Nausea (antiemetic)
Propacet	Pain management (narcotic analgesic)
Propecia	Hair loss
propoxyphene	Pain management (narcotic analgesic)
propranolol	High blood pressure, heart problems, angina (beta blocker)
Proscar	Prostate enlargement
Protonix	Gastric problems
Proventil	Breathing problems (bronchodilator)
Provera	Gynecologic problems (progestogen)
Provigil	Narcolepsy
Prozac	Depression (antidepressant)
Pulmicort	Asthma
Pyridium	Urinary tract infections, pain
Quinaglute	Ventricular arrhythmias (antiarrhythmic)
quinapril	High blood pressure (ACE inhibitor)
Qvar	Asthma, breathing problems (anti-inflammatory)
ramipril	High blood pressure (ACE inhibitor)
ranitidine	Ulcers, gastric problems (antiulcer)
Reglan	Nausea (antiemetic)
Relafen	Inflammation, pain (anti-inflammatory)
Remeron	Anxiety, depression (sedative)
Restoril	Sleep disorders (hypnotic)
Retrovir	Antiretroviral
Risperdal	Psychological disorders (antipsychotic)

Ritalin	Attention deficit disorder, narcolepsy
Robaxin	Muscle spasms (muscle relaxant)
Roxicet	Pain management (narcotic analgesic)
Rythmol	Heart problems, ventricular tachycardia
Sectral	High blood pressure (beta blocker)
Septra	Infection (antibiotic)
Serevent	Asthma, breathing problems (bronchodilators)
Seroquel	Psychological disorders (antipsychotic)
sertraline	Depression (antidepressant)
Serzone	Depression (antidepressant)
simvastatin	High cholesterol
Sinemet	Parkinson's disease (anti-Parkinson)
Sinequan	Anxiety, depression (antidepressant)
Singulair	Asthma
Skelaxin	Muscle relaxant
Slo-Bid	Breathing problems, asthma (bronchodilator)
Slow-K	Potassium replacement, taken with diuretics
Soma	Muscle spasms (muscle relaxant)
Spiriva	Breathing problems
spironolactone	High blood pressure, heart failure (diuretic)
Suboxone	Treatment of opioid dependence
sucralfate	Ulcers (antiulcer)
Sular	High blood pressure
sulfamethoxazole	Infection (antibiotic)
sulfasalazine	Ulcerative colitis (antibacterial)
sulfisoxazole	Infection (antibiotic)
Sumycin	Infection (antibiotic)
Suprax	Infection (antibiotic)
Sustiva	Antiretroviral

continues

Symbicort	Asthma
Synthroid	Thyroid disease (thyroid hormone)
Tagamet	Ulcers, gastric problems (antiulcer)
Tamiflu	Antiviral
tamoxifen	Cancer (antineoplastic)
Tavist	Allergies (antihistamine)
Tegretol	Seizure disorder (anticonvulsant)
temazepam	Insomnia (sedative)
Tenex	High blood pressure (alpha blocker)
Tenormin	High blood pressure, heart problems, angina (beta blocker)
Tequin	Infection (anti-infective)
terazosin	High blood pressure (alpha blocker)
tetracycline	Infection (antibiotic)
Theo-Dur	Breathing problems (bronchodilator)
theophylline	Breathing problems (bronchodilator)
Tiazac	High blood pressure
Ticlid	Stroke (antiplatelet)
Tigan	Nausea and vomiting (antiemetic)
Tofranil	Depression (antidepressant)
Tolinase	Diabetes (oral antidiabetic)
Topamax	Seizures
Toprol	High blood pressure (beta blocker)
Toradol	Short-term pain
tramadol	Pain (analgesic)
trazodone	Depression (antidepressant)
Trental	Vascular disease (blood thinner)
triamterene	High blood pressure (diuretic)
Triavil	Anxiety, depression (antidepressant)
Tricor	High triglycerides (antilipemic)
trimethoprim	Infection, mainly urinary tract (antibiotic)
Trimox	Infection (antibiotic)

Triphasil	Birth control pill
Trivora-28	Birth control pills
Tussionex	Cough (antitussive)
Tylenol with codeine (Tylenol #3)	Pain
Ultram	Pain (analgesic)
valacyclovir	Herpes (antiviral)
Valium	Anxiety (antianxiety)
valproic acid	Seizure disorder (anticonvulsant)
Valtrex	Herpes (antiviral)
Vantin	Infections (antibiotic)
Vasotec	High blood pressure, heart failure
Veetids	Infection (antibiotic)
venlafaxine	Depression (antidepressant)
Ventolin	Breathing problems (bronchodilator)
verapamil	Angina, high blood pressure, rapid heart rate
Viagra	Male impotence
Vibramycin	Infection (antibiotic)
Vicodin	Pain (narcotic)
Vicoprofen	Pain (narcotic analgesic)
Viramune	Antiretroviral
Viread	Antiretroviral
Voltaren	Arthritis (anti-inflammatory)
Vytorin	High cholesterol
warfarin sodium	Blood clots (blood thinner)
Wellbutrin	Depression (antidepressant)
Xalatan	Glaucoma
Xanax	Anxiety, depression (sedative)
Xenical	Weight loss
Xopenex	Breathing problems
Yasmin	Birth control
YAZ	Birth control

continues

Zantac	Ulcers, gastric problems (antiulcer)
Zerit	Antiretroviral
Zestoretic	High blood pressure
Zestril	High blood pressure (ACE inhibitor)
Zetia	High cholesterol
Ziac	High blood pressure (beta blocker, diuretic)
Zithromax	Infection (antibiotic)
Zocor	High cholesterol (cholesterol-lowering agent)
Zofran	Nausea
Zoloft	Depression (antidepressant)
zolpidem	Sleep aid
Zomig	Migraine headaches
zonisamide	Seizures
Zovirax	Herpes, shingles, chicken pox (antiviral)
Zyflo	Asthma
Zyloprim	Gout
Zyprexa	Psychological disorders (antipsychotic)
Zyrtec	Allergies (antihistamine)

New Jersey Poison Control Center Information and Education System

Hotline

A national number to reach poison control centers **(1-800-222-1222)** provides free, 24-hour professional poison expertise and treatment advice. All calls are answered by pharmacists, physicians, and nurses who are toxicology specialists.

Information and Education

New Jersey Poison Information and Education System (NJPIES) is designated as one of 57 U.S. regional poison control centers nationwide and is New Jersey's only poison control center. Visit **www.njpies.org** for more information.

A poison is any substance that can harm your body, make you sick, or even kill you if used in the wrong way, by the wrong person, in the wrong amount. Most poisonings involve household items such as medicines, cleaning supplies, cosmetics, and personal care items, but they may also be caused by alcohol, recreational drugs, medications, food, or plants.

Poisoning can be classified according to the way the poison enters the body. The four primary routes are:

- Ingestion
- Inhalation
- Injection
- Absorption

Ingestion

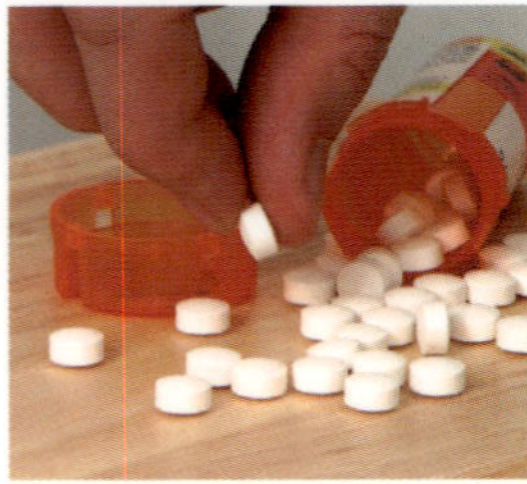

Ingestion occurs when poison enters the body through the mouth and is absorbed by the digestive system. Signs and symptoms of ingested poisons include the following:

- Unusual breath odors
- Discoloration or burning around the mouth
- Nausea and/or vomiting
- Abdominal pain
- Diarrhea

Inhalation

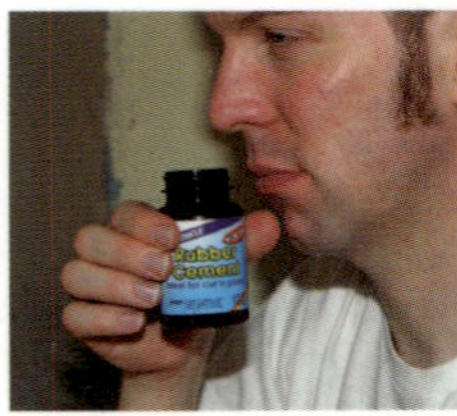

Inhalation occurs when a poison enters the body through the mouth or nose and is absorbed by mucous membranes lining the respiratory system. Signs and symptoms of inhaled poisons include the following:

- Respiratory distress
- Dizziness
- Cough
- Headache
- Hoarseness
- Confusion
- Chest pain

Injection

Injection occurs when a poison enters the body through a small opening in the skin and spreads through the circulatory system. Injection can occur as a result of an insect sting or the intentional use of a hypodermic needle to inject a poisonous substance into the body. Signs and symptoms of injected poisons include the following:

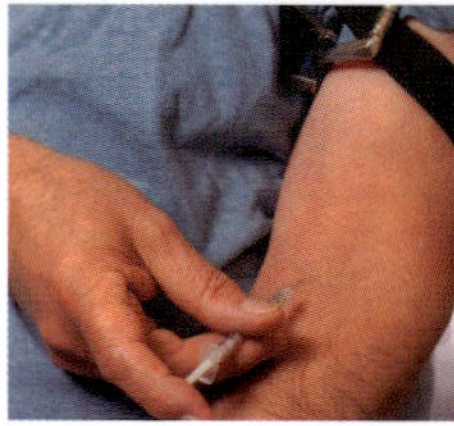

- Obvious injury site
- Tenderness
- Swelling
- Red streaks radiating from injection site
- Weakness
- Dizziness
- Localized pain
- Itching

Absorption

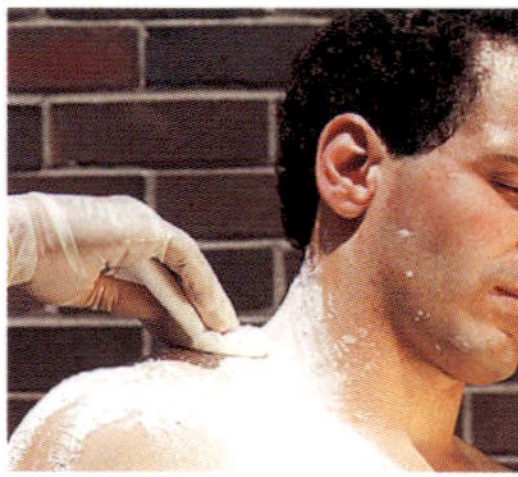

Absorption occurs when a poison enters the body through intact skin and spreads through the circulatory system. Signs and symptoms of absorbed poisons include the following:

- Traces of powder or liquid on the skin
- Inflammation or redness of the skin
- Chemical burns
- Rash
- Burning
- Itching
- Nausea and vomiting
- Dizziness
- Shock

Phone Numbers and Radio Frequencies

General

Use the spaces provided to fill in your local phone numbers.

TABLE 1 Useful Phone Numbers

Adult Protective Services (APS)	*1-800-792-8820
AIDS Information	1-800-624-2377
Air Medical Unit (AMU)	1-800-332-4356
Alzheimer's Information	1-609-943-4985
American Red Cross	____________
Animal Control	____________
Battered Women's Hotline	1-800-572-SAFE (7233)
CHEMTREC	1-800-262-8200
Child Abuse/Neglect	1-877-NJ-ABUSE (65-22873)
CISM Team	1-877-294-HELP (4357)
Communications/Dispatch	____________
Domestic Violence Center	1-800-572-7233
Elder Abuse/Neglect	1-877-582-6995
Hazardous Materials Team	1-609-633-1418
NJ State Health and Senior Services Department	1-800-367-6543
County Health Dept	____________
Local Health Dept	____________
Homeless Shelter	____________

Hospital Complaints	1-800-792-9770
Infection Control	__________
MedicAlert Emergency Response	1-800-625-3780 or 1-209-634-4917
NJ State Medical Examiner/Coroner	1-609-896-8900
NJ Office of Emergency Medical Services (OEMS)	1-609-633-7777
Poison/Drug Information Center	1-800-222-1222
Psychiatric Emergency Services	__________
Rape/Sexual Abuse Crisis Center	__________
Regional Emergency Management Communications Systems (REMCS)	
Emergency lines	1-973-972-0911 or 1-973-973-7000
Nonemergency lines	1-800-631-3444 or 1-973-972-6290
SIDS Hotline	1-800-545-7437
Stress Response Team	1-866-4U-NJ-1ST (48-65-178)
Suicide Prevention Hotline	1-800-273-TALK (8255)
Terrorism Reporting	1-866-4-SAFE-NJ (7233-65)
Towing Service/Heavy Wrecker	__________
Translators (note language)	__________
Youth Hotline	1-888-222-2228
__________	__________
__________	__________

continues

*Note: There is an APS program in each of the 21 counties that is monitored and evaluated by state staff. See the *Abuse and Neglect* protocol for phone numbers by county.

Mobile Intensive Care Units (MICU)

Also known as Advanced Life Support (ALS)

TABLE 2 MICU Contact Information

County/MICU Name(s)	MICU Telephone
Atlantic	
AtlantiCare—MICU 6685 Washington Avenue Egg Harbor Township NJ 08234	(609) 407-6360
Bergen	
Englewood Hospital & Medical Center—MICU 350 Engle Street Englewood NJ 07631	(201) 894-3416
Hackensack University Medical Center—MICU 30 Prospect Avenue Hackensack NJ 07601	(201) 678-1601
Holy Name Hospital—MICU 718 Teaneck Road Teaneck NJ 07666	(201) 541-6322

The Valley Hospital—MICU 233 North VanDien Avenue Ridgewood NJ 07450	(201) 447-8447
Burlington	
Virtua Health Emergency Medical Services 523 Fellowship Road, Suite 270 Mt. Laurel NJ 08054	(856) 581-7500
Camden	
Virtua Health Emergency Medical Services 523 Fellowship Road, Suite 270 Mt. Laurel NJ 08054	(856) 581-7500
Cape May	
AtlantiCare—MICU 6685 Washington Avenue Egg Harbor Township NJ 08234	(609) 407-6360
Cumberland	
Underwood Memorial Hospital-MICU 238 South Evergreen Avenue Woodbury NJ 08096	(856) 384-1000
Essex	
MONOC-MICU 4806 Megill Road Neptune NJ 07753	(732) 929-3045
Atlantic Health System-Mountainside 22 Claremont Avenue Montclair NJ 07042	(908) 522-2865
University Hospital EMS-MICU 150 Cabinet Street Newark NJ 07107	(973) 972-4850

continues

TABLE 2 MICU Contact Information, continued

County/MICU Name(s)	MICU Director/Telephone
Gloucester	
Underwood Memorial Hospital-MICU 238 South Evergreen Avenue Woodbury NJ 08096	(856) 384-1000
Hudson	
Jersey City Medical Center-MICU 415 Montgomery Street Jersey City NJ 07302	(201) 547-6107
Hunterdon	
Hunterdon Medical Center-MICU 2100 Wescott Drive Flemington NJ 08822	(908) 788-2500
Mercer	
Capital Health System 65 Prospect St. Trenton NJ 08618	(609) 394-4516
Middlesex	
Solaris Health System-MICU 65 James Street Edison NJ 08818	(908) 668-2928
Raritan Bay Medical Center-MICU 530 New Brunswick Avenue Perth Amboy NJ 08861	(732) 324-5093
Robert Wood Johnson University Hospital-MICU 126 Paterson Street New Brunswick NJ 08901	(732) 937-8728

Monmouth

MONOC-MICU (732) 929-3045
4806 Megill Road
Neptune NJ 07753

Morris

Chilton Memorial Hospital-MICU (973) 831-5170
97 West Parkway
Pompton Plains NJ 07444

Atlantic Health System-Morristown-MICU (908) 522-2865
100 Madison Avenue
Morristown NJ 07962

St. Clare's Hospital/Dover-MICU (973) 537-5654
400 West Blackwell Street
Dover NJ 07801

MONOC-MICU (732) 929-3045
4806 Megill Road
Neptune NJ 07753

Passaic

St. Joseph's Regional Medical Center-MICU (973) 754-2262
703 Main Street
Paterson NJ 07503

MONOC-MICU (732) 929-3045
4806 Megill Road
Neptune NJ 07753

Salem

Underwood Memorial Hospital-MICU (856) 384-1000
238 South Evergreen Avenue
Woodbury NJ 08096

continues

Somerset

Somerset Medical Center-MICU 110 Rehill Avenue Somerville NJ 08876	(908) 203-6253

Sussex

St. Clare's Hospital/Dover-MICU 400 West Blackwell Street Dover NJ 07801	(973) 537-5654

Union

Solaris Health System-MICU 65 James Street Edison NJ 08818	(908) 668-2928
Atlantic Health System-Overlook-MICU 99 Beauvoir Avenue Summit NJ 07901	(908) 522-2865
RWJ University Hospital-Rahway-MICU 865 Stone Street Rahway NJ 07065	(732) 499-6005
Trinitas Hospital-MICU 425 Morris Avenue Elizabeth NJ 07202	(908) 994-8644
MONOC-MICU 4806 Megill Road Neptune NJ 07753	(732) 929-3045

Warren

Hunterdon Medical Center-MICU 2100 Wescott Drive Flemington NJ 08822	(908) 788-2500
St. Clare's Hospital/Dover-MICU 400 West Blackwell Street Dover NJ 07801	(973) 537-5654

REMCS Radio Channels

Mobile and portable radios are required on the JEMS systems for all licensed ALS and BLS providers. The four channels are determined as follows:

- **JEMS 1:** Local dispatch; primary channel used to communicate to local dispatch center, regardless of frequency band.
- **JEMS 2:** 155.340 MHz CSQ; ambulance to hospital ED.
- **JEMS 3:** 155.280 MHz CSQ; statewide EMS coordination.
- **JEMS 4:** 153.785 MHz 131.8 TX only same as SPEN 4; statewide mobile public safety coordination.

Interoperability

New Jersey EMS agencies will utilize the national/state interoperability radio system to communicate with responding agencies as necessary to communicate during emergencies:

- VCALL Interoperability Call Channel—155.7525.
- VTAC1 Interoperability Tactical Channel—151.1375.
- VTAC2 Interoperability Tactical Channel—154.4525.
- VTAC3 Interoperability Tactical Channel—158.7375.
- VTAC4 Interoperability Tactical Channel—159.4725.
- All VTAC radio system frequencies will utilize Nationwide CTCSS 156.7.

Hospital Phone Numbers and Radio Channels

Hospital Name	Medical Control Phone Number	Emergency Room Phone Number	Medical Control Radio Channel

Hospital Phone Numbers and Radio Channels

Hospital Name	Medical Control Phone Number	Emergency Room Phone Number	Medical Control Radio Channel

Stress Management

Prevention and Planning

Proactive stress management is essential to the provision of emergency response workers. Successful stress management is built on prevention and planning, a solid understanding of roles and responsibilities, support from colleagues, good self-care, and seeking help when needed.

Self-Care

The Substance Abuse and Mental Health Services Administration (SAMHSA) recommends "10 Things to Do Each Day" for self-care in the face of difficult work.

1. Get enough sleep.
2. Eat enough healthy food.
3. Vary the work that you do.
4. Do some light exercise.
5. Do something pleasurable.
6. Focus on what you did well.
7. Learn from your mistakes.
8. Share a private joke.
9. Pray, meditate, or relax.
10. Support a colleague.

During Deployments

Individuals and teams can take several steps to reduce stress during deployments:

1. Adhere to established safety policies and procedures.
2. Seek and offer support to coworkers.
3. Take regular breaks whenever you experience troubling incidents and after each work shift.
4. Avoid alcohol, tobacco, drugs, and excessive caffeine.

5. Rotate work between low- and high-stress activities.
6. Rotate work from the scene to routine assignments, as practical.
7. Limit on-duty work hours to no more than 12 hours per day.
8. Call home daily.

After a Deployment

Trained counselors through the Mental Health Association in New Jersey are available to talk to you. The toll free confidential helpline is **1-877-294-HELP (4357)** or TTY number **1-877-294-4356.**

Critical incident stress management (CISM) is a process developed to address acute stress situations and potentially decrease the likelihood that post-traumatic stress disorder will develop after a stressful event.

Following a disaster response it is not uncommon to experience physical and emotional fatigue. It is helpful to take time to stop and reflect on the experience and how it has changed you. You can help manage your stress after the crisis by:

1. Participating in stress management activities with coworkers.
2. Reconnecting with your family.
3. Having a physical checkup, if indicated.
4. Continuing normal leisure activities; staying involved with hobbies and interests.
5. Using stress management and relaxation techniques such as exercise, meditation, acupuncture, and massage therapy.
6. Drawing upon already existing religious (spirituality) beliefs.
7. Avoiding use of alcohol, tobacco, or drugs to cope with stress.
8. Seeking out professional assistance, if necessary.

Self-Monitoring for Signs of Stress

Be familiar with signs of too much stress. Self-awareness involves recognizing and heeding early warning signs of stress reactions. A buddy system, where coworkers agree to observe one another's stress reactions, can be important. Signs that you may need stress management assistance include the following:

1. Disorientation or confusion and difficulty communicating thoughts.
2. Difficulty remembering instructions.
3. Difficulty maintaining balance.
4. Becoming easily frustrated and being uncharacteristically argumentative.
5. Tearfulness, uncontrolled crying.
6. Inability to engage in problem-solving and difficulty making decisions.
7. Unnecessary risk-taking.
8. Tremors, headaches, or nausea.
9. Visual or auditory distortion.
10. Colds or flulike symptoms.
11. Limited attention span and difficulty concentrating.
12. Loss of objectivity.
13. Inability to relax when off duty.
14. Refusal to follow orders or to leave the scene.
15. Increased use of drugs/alcohol.
16. Unusual clumsiness, decreased coordination.

Source: Adapted from the US Department of Health and Human Services (DHHS) Substance Abuse Mental Health Services Administration (SAMHSA), "Caring for Yourself in the Face of Difficult Work," created in cooperation with Idaho State University.

Vehicle Safety Reminders

1. The crewmember who is operating an emergency vehicle must possess a valid driver's license. The license must be made available to OEMS staff upon request.
2. All crewmembers must carry valid/original certification cards as well as photo ID. These must be made available to OEMS staff upon request.
3. Crewmembers must be familiar with the proper operation of the EMS communication equipment.
4. All emergency vehicles must be locked and inaccessible to anyone other than the crew members when unattended.
5. Check expiration dates on a monthly basis on all supplies and equipment.
6. Ensure that all biomedical equipment is operating properly and in accordance with manufacturer's recommendations (example: AED).
7. Ensure that the vehicle air conditioning and heating systems are working properly.
8. All interior surfaces of the vehicle must be impervious to blood, vomitus, grease, oil, and common cleaning materials.
9. All equipment and supplies must be stored in a crashworthy manner. No items are to be left unsecured on countertops or on top of shelves.
10. Ensure that all cabinets have a properly working positive-action latch in place.
11. All stretcher mattresses and seat covers must be in good condition and have no tears present.
12. Check at the beginning of every shift that all emergency lights and sirens are working properly.
13. Ensure that *No Smoking* signs are present in the driver and passenger compartments.
14. Ensure that all vehicle seat belts are present and working properly.
15. Ensure that all bench seat latches are working properly.

16. Ensure that the fire extinguisher is fully charged and secured in a commercially designed quick release bracket.
17. Ensure that the vehicle exhaust system and gaskets around the exterior doors and windows are in good condition.
18. The vehicle must have a current Motor Vehicle Commission (MVC) Inspection decal (ambulances are NOT EXEMPT from MVC Inspections).
19. Ensure that the vehicle has a current/valid registration and insurance card.
20. The vehicle must meet current certification requirements of the applicable paragraphs of the Federal KKK-A-1822 Federal Motor Vehicle Safety Standards (FMVSS), as amended and supplemented. Must have FMVSS "Star of Life" vehicle certification label affixed to vehicle.
21. The vehicle must be tagged by the vehicle manufacturer or converter.
22. The vehicle must have a passive barrier at the forward end of the bench seat.
23. Routinely check the main oxygen system to ensure that the straps/frame are properly secured.
24. Portable oxygen cylinders must be properly secured in a commercially approved holder. Velcro and hook and loop type devices are not considered crashworthy.
25. On-board oxygen retention systems must meet the "Ambulance Manufacturers Division" (AMD) standards as reported by the (FMVSS). The following are basic guidelines established by the Office of Emergency Medical Services.
    - Three points of restraint on the cylinder; the bottom two restraints must not be "quick release"-type buckles.
    - A "yoke"-type restraint is acceptable as one point on the top of the cylinder.
    - Bracketed/frame-type enclosure.
    - The oxygen cylinder controls shall be accessible from inside the vehicle.
26. Ensure that portable and on-board suction devices have all components present and are fully charged and operational.

27. Doorway openings shall not be obstructed and must comply with FMVSS specifications.
28. Interior door handles shall be accessible and not obstructed (e.g., by cabinetry, accessories, etc.).
29. All glass must be intact and free of cracks.
30. Exhaust systems must be secured and free of damage and leaks. Exhaust pipe must extend beyond the doors and the edge of the vehicle body.
31. Air bag deployment zones should be void of accessories (MDTs, GPSs, lights, etc.).